EPI COOKBOOK FOR NEWLY DIAGNOSED 2024

Culinary Wellness: Nourishing Recipes for Vibrant Living

Benjamin Leon

Copyright © 2024

All Rights Are Reserved

The content in this book may not be reproduced, duplicated, or transferred without the express written permission of the author or publisher. Under no circumstances will the publisher or author be held liable or legally responsible for any losses, expenditures, or damages incurred directly or indirectly as a consequence of the information included in this book.

Legal Remarks

Copyright protection applies to this publication. It is only intended for personal use. No piece of this work may be modified, distributed, sold, quoted, or paraphrased without the author's or publisher's consent.

Disclaimer Statement

Please keep in mind that the contents of this booklet are meant for educational and recreational purposes. Every effort has been made to offer accurate, up-to-date, reliable, and thorough information. There are, however, no stated or implied assurances of any kind. Readers understand that the author is providing competent counsel. The content in this book originates from several sources. Please seek the opinion of a competent professional before using any of the tactics outlined in this book. By reading this book, the reader agrees that the author will not be held accountable for any direct or indirect damages resulting from the use of the information contained therein, including, but not limited to, errors, omissions, or inaccuracies.

Table of Contents

- INTRODUCTION 1
- UNDERSTANDING EPI: WHAT YOU NEED TO KNOW 4
  - What is Exocrine Pancreatic Insufficiency (EPI)? 4
  - Causes and Symptoms 5
  - Diagnosis and Treatment Options 6
- EPI-FRIENDLY EATING BASICS 8
  - Adapting Your Diet to Manage EPI 8
  - Importance of Enzyme Replacement Therapy (ERT) 8
  - Key Nutrients and Dietary Considerations 9
  - Meal Planning Tips for EPI 10
  - Essential Kitchen Tools and Ingredients 10
  - Must-Have Kitchen Equipment 11
  - Pantry Staples for EPI-Friendly Cooking 11
- BEYOND THE BASICS 14
  - Advanced Cooking Techniques for EPI-Friendly Meals 14
  - Cooking for Multiple Dietary Restrictions 15
  - International Flavors Made EPI-Friendly 16
  - Tips for Dining Out with EPI 17
- BREAKFAST RECIPES 18
  - EPI-Friendly Veggie Omelet 18

EPI-Friendly Banana Oat Pancakes 19

EPI-Friendly Greek Yogurt Parfait 20

EPI-Friendly Avocado Toast 21

EPI-Friendly Berry Smoothie Bowl 22

Soothing Banana Porridge 23

Savory Spinach and Mushroom Scramble 24

Ginger Turmeric Smoothie 25

Quinoa Breakfast Bowl 26

Energizing Chia Seed Pudding 27

Hearty Quinoa Breakfast Bowl 28

Energizing Chia Seed Pudding 30

Zesty Spinach and Egg Muffins 31

Soothing Banana Porridge 32

Savory Sweet Potato Hash 33

Protein-Packed Scrambled Tofu 34

Oatmeal Breakfast Cookies 35

Egg and Veggie Breakfast Burrito 37

Creamy Coconut Chia Pudding 38

Berry Banana Smoothie Bowl 39

SNACKS RECIPES 41

Nutty Energy Bites 41

Avocado Toast with Tomato and Basil 42

Greek Yogurt Parfait 43

Hummus and Veggie Stuffed Pita Pockets 44

Vegetable Sushi Rolls 45

Crunchy Chickpea Snack 46

Apple and Peanut Butter Rice Cakes 47

Vegetable Crudité with Hummus 48

Quinoa and Black Bean Salad Cups 49

Banana Almond Butter Bites 50

Zesty Cucumber Hummus Cups 51

Crispy Baked Kale Chips 52

Sweet Potato Toasts with Almond Butter 53

Mango Salsa with Whole Grain Crackers 54

Quinoa-Stuffed Bell Pepper 55

Nutty Banana Oat Bars 57

Roasted Chickpea Trail Mix 58

Greek Yogurt Berry Parfait 59

Stuffed Celery Sticks 60

Turkey and Avocado Roll-Ups 61

DESSERTS RECIPES 63

Banana Almond Chia Pudding 63

Avocado Chocolate Mousse 64

Coconut Mango Rice Pudding 65

Baked Apples with Cinnamon and Walnuts 66

Frozen Berry Yogurt Bark 67

Chia Seed Pudding with Berries 69

Baked Apple Chips 70

Coconut Banana Ice Cream 71

Chocolate Avocado Mousse 72

Cinnamon Baked Pears 73

Coconut Chia Pudding with Fresh Fruit 74

Almond Flour Banana Bread 75

Baked Coconut Mango Oatmeal Cups 77

Chocolate Peanut Butter Protein Balls 78

Apple Cinnamon Quinoa Breakfast Bars 79

Berry Avocado Parfait 81

Pumpkin Spice Chia Seed Pudding 82

Coconut Mango Rice Pudding 83

Dark Chocolate Avocado Mousse 84

Banana Oatmeal Cookies 85

SOUP RECIPES 88

Creamy Butternut Squash Soup 88

Lentil and Vegetable Soup 89

Roasted Tomato Basil Soup 91

Ginger Carrot Soup 92

Creamy Mushroom Soup 94

Spicy Black Bean Soup 95

Butternut Squash Soup 97

Lentil Soup 98

Tomato Basil Soup 100

Carrot Ginger Soup 101

Spinach and Potato Soup 103

Vegetable Quinoa Soup 104

Creamy Cauliflower Soup 106

Lentil and Vegetable Soup 107

Butternut Squash Soup 109

Tomato Basil Soup 110

Chicken and Vegetable Soup 112

Lentil and Spinach Soup 113

Butternut Squash Soup 114

Mushroom Barley Soup 116

Tomato and White Bean Soup 117

SEAFOOD RECIPES 119

Grilled Lemon Herb Salmon 119

Baked Lemon Garlic Shrimp 120

Seared Scallops with Garlic Butter 121

Grilled Shrimp Skewers 122

Pan-Seared Halibut with Lemon Herb Sauce 123

Cajun Grilled Shrimp Tacos 125

Baked Lemon Garlic Cod 126

Coconut Shrimp Curry 127

Lemon Garlic Butter Scallops 129

Grilled Salmon with Dill Sauce 130

Grilled Lemon Herb Salmon 131

Lemon Garlic Shrimp Pasta 132

Baked Lemon Dill Cod 133

Garlic Butter Scallops 135

Lemon Herb Tilapia 136

Lemon Garlic Grilled Shrimp 137

Baked Salmon with Dill 138

Garlic Butter Lobster Tails 139

Tuna Salad Lettuce Wraps 140

Grilled Swordfish with Mango Salsa 141

SMOOTHIE RECIPES 143

Berry Blast Smoothie 143

Tropical Paradise Smoothie 144

Green Goddess Smoothie 144

Protein Power Smoothie 145

Coconut Kale Smoothie 146

Tropical Green Smoothie 147

Berry Spinach Smoothie 148

Creamy Avocado Smoothie 149

Peanut Butter Banana Smoothie 150

Blueberry Almond Smoothie 151

Berry Blast Smoothie 151

Green Goddess Smoothie 152

Tropical Paradise Smoothie 153

Creamy Berry Smoothie 154

Chocolate Peanut Butter Smoothie 155

Green Detox Smoothie 156

Berry Blast Smoothie 157

Tropical Paradise Smoothie 158

Creamy Peanut Butter Banana Smoothie 159

Vanilla Almond Protein Smoothie 159

MEAL PLAN 161

Day 1 161
Day 2 161
Day 3 161
Day 4 161
Day 5 161
Day 6 162
Day 7 162
Day 8 162
Day 9 162
Day 10 162
Day 11 162
Day 12 163
Day 13 163
Day 14 163
Day 15 163
Day 16 163
Day 17 164
Day 18 164
Day 19 164
Day 20 164
Day 21 164

CONCLUSION 166

INTRODUCTION

Welcome, dear reader, to the culinary journey of a lifetime. But first, let's address the elephant in the room or should I say, the pancreas-shaped mascot sitting at our dinner table? Yes, I'm talking about Exocrine Pancreatic Insufficiency, or EPI for short. If you're holding this book, chances are you've recently been diagnosed with EPI, and you're likely feeling a whirlwind of emotions right now. Confusion, frustration, perhaps even a dash of fear mixed in with a sprinkle of uncertainty. Don't worry; you're not alone.

Before we dive headfirst into the world of EPI-friendly cooking, let me introduce myself. I'm your culinary guide, your kitchen companion, and your fellow EPI navigator. My name is [Benjamin Leon], and like you, I've walked the winding path of pancreatic insufficiency. I know the frustration of trying to decipher what's safe to eat, the disappointment of missing out on beloved dishes, and the occasional (okay, frequent) grumbling of a not-so-happy tummy. But fear not, dear reader, for I'm here to tell you that delicious, satisfying meals are still within reach no, scratch that within arm's reach. We're going to tackle EPI one recipe at a time, armed with a spoon, a spatula, and a whole lot of culinary courage. Now, you might be wondering why on earth we're making a big fuss about food when your pancreas seems to be playing a game of hide-and-seek. Well, here's the scoop: what you put on your plate matters a lot. With EPI, your body doesn't produce enough digestive enzymes to break down food properly, leading to a whole host of digestive woes. But fear not, my hungry friend, for we have a secret weapon in our arsenal: the power of food. By crafting meals specifically tailored to EPI, we can help ease digestive discomfort, boost nutrient absorption, and reignite your love affair with eating.

In this cookbook, you'll find a treasure trove of EPI-friendly recipes designed to tantalize your taste buds while keeping your pancreas happy. But before we jump into the kitchen and start wielding spatulas like culinary wizards, let's lay down some groundwork. In the opening chapters, we'll unravel the mysteries of EPI, exploring everything from its sneaky symptoms to the best ways to manage it through diet. Consider it your crash course in all things pancreas-related, minus the boring medical jargon and the intimidating diagrams.

Once we've got our EPI basics down pat, it's time to roll up our sleeves and get cooking. From breakfast delights to dinner feasts, from snack attacks to sweet treats, we've got every meal of the day covered EPI style. Think mouthwatering smoothies that'll put a pep in your step, hearty stews that'll warm you from the inside out, and decadent desserts that'll satisfy your sweet tooth without sending your pancreas into a panic. And fear not, my gluten-free, dairy-free, vegan, and vegetarian friends—there's a little something for everyone in these pages.

But this cookbook isn't just about feeding your body; it's about nourishing your soul. It's about reclaiming the joy of cooking, the pleasure of sharing a meal with loved ones, and the satisfaction of knowing that you're taking control of your health one delicious bite at a time. So go ahead, dear reader, grab a fork, and let's embark on this culinary adventure together. Whether you're a seasoned chef or a kitchen newbie, whether you're cooking for one or feeding a crowd, there's a place for you at our table.

Before we part ways and dive into the deliciousness that awaits, let me leave you with one final thought: living with EPI might have its challenges, but it also has its silver linings. It's a reminder to savor each bite, to appreciate the simple pleasures of a well-cooked meal, and to cherish the moments spent gathered around the table with the ones we love. So here's to good food, good company, and good health. Let's eat!

With love and ladles,

UNDERSTANDING EPI: WHAT YOU NEED TO KNOW

Exocrine Pancreatic Insufficiency (EPI) is a complex condition that affects the digestive system, specifically the pancreas—an organ often underestimated in its importance until it starts causing trouble. But fear not, dear reader, for I'm here to shed some light on this often misunderstood ailment. So grab a comfy seat and a cup of tea (or whatever beverage tickles your fancy), and let's dive into the fascinating world of EPI.

What is Exocrine Pancreatic Insufficiency (EPI)?

To put it simply, Exocrine Pancreatic Insufficiency, or EPI, is a condition where the pancreas fails to produce enough digestive enzymes to properly break down food in the small intestine. Now, you might be wondering, "What's the big deal about digestive enzymes anyway?" Well, my curious friend, let me tell you they're kind of a big deal.

You see, digestive enzymes are like the culinary wizards of your digestive system. They're responsible for breaking down fats, proteins, and carbohydrates into smaller, more absorbable molecules that your body can then use for energy and nourishment. Without enough enzymes, your body struggles to digest food properly, leading to a whole host of unpleasant symptoms like bloating, gas, diarrhea, and malnutrition. Not exactly a walk in the park, huh?

So why does this enzyme shortage happen in the first place? Ah, that's where things get a tad more complicated. EPI can be caused by a variety of factors, ranging from medical conditions to lifestyle choices. For some folks, it's a result of chronic pancreatitis a condition characterized by inflammation of the pancreas due to long-term alcohol abuse, gallstones, or other factors. In others, it might be linked to cystic fibrosis, a genetic disorder that affects the production of mucus and digestive enzymes in the body. And then there are those unlucky souls who develop EPI for no apparent reason at all a frustrating reality that highlights just how mysterious and unpredictable our bodies can be.

But fear not, my puzzled pal, for understanding the causes of EPI is only half the battle. The other half? Recognizing the symptoms that accompany this pesky pancreas problem.

Causes and Symptoms

Let's start with the symptoms, shall we? Picture this: you've just finished a delicious meal a hearty plate of pasta, perhaps, or a sizzling steak fresh off the grill. But instead of feeling satisfied and content, you're left feeling bloated, uncomfortable, and downright miserable. Sound familiar? If so, you might be experiencing some of the telltale signs of EPI.

One of the most common symptoms of EPI is chronic diarrhea a delightful little side effect of undigested food making its hasty exit from your body. But that's not all; bloating, gas, abdominal pain, and unexplained weight loss are also frequent companions on this digestive rollercoaster ride. And let's not forget about the not-so-pleasant aroma that often accompanies these digestive woes a delightful reminder that our bodies are anything but subtle when it comes to sending distress signals.

Now, you might be thinking, "But wait, couldn't these symptoms be caused by a myriad of other digestive issues?" And you'd be absolutely right! That's what makes diagnosing EPI a bit of a puzzle one that often requires the keen eye (and sharp wit) of a medical professional.

Diagnosis and Treatment Options

So, how does one go about diagnosing this elusive EPI creature? Well, my friend, it typically involves a combination of medical history, physical exams, and a few nifty tests thrown into the mix. Your doctor might start by asking about your symptoms, you're eating habits, and any existing medical conditions you might have. From there, they might perform a physical exam to check for signs of malnutrition or abdominal tenderness.

But the real magic happens when they whip out their secret weapon: diagnostic tests. These can include blood tests to measure levels of digestive enzymes in your bloodstream, stool tests to check for undigested fat, and imaging tests like CT scans or MRIs to get a closer look at your pancreas. It's like playing detective, only instead of solving crimes, we're solving digestive mysteries.

Once you've got that elusive EPI diagnosis in hand, it's time to talk treatment options. And lucky for you, there are plenty to choose from! One of the most common treatments for EPI is enzyme replacement therapy (ERT) a fancy way of saying that we're going to give your digestive system a helping hand by providing it with the enzymes it so desperately needs. These enzymes usually come in the form of capsules or tablets that you take with meals, helping to break down food and alleviate those pesky digestive symptoms.

But that's not the only trick up our sleeves. In addition to ERT, your doctor might recommend dietary changes to help ease digestive discomfort and improve nutrient absorption. This might involve avoiding certain foods that are high in fat or difficult to digest, opting for smaller, more frequent meals throughout the day, and making sure you're getting plenty of water and other fluids to stay hydrated. It's all about finding what works best for you and your body a bit of trial and error, if you will.

And let's not forget about the importance of self-care in managing EPI. Stress, lack of sleep, and poor lifestyle habits can all exacerbate digestive symptoms, so it's crucial to prioritize your overall health and well-being. That means getting plenty of rest, finding healthy ways to manage stress, and making time for activities that bring you joy and relaxation. After all, a happy pancreas is a healthy pancreas!

So there you have it, dear reader a crash course in all things EPI. From its sneaky causes to its not-so-subtle symptoms, and from diagnosis to treatment options, we've covered it all. But remember, knowledge is power, and armed with the right information and a sprinkle of culinary know-how, you can take control of your digestive destiny and start living your best (and most delicious) life. So go ahead, my intrepid friend, dig in, and don't let EPI hold you back from enjoying every mouthful. After all, life's too short to let a cranky pancreas cramp your style

EPI-FRIENDLY EATING BASICS

Welcome to the heart of our culinary journey EPI-Friendly Eating Basics. In this chapter, we'll delve into the essentials of managing Exocrine Pancreatic Insufficiency (EPI) through diet and lifestyle adjustments. So grab a seat at the table and let's explore how you can nourish your body while keeping your pancreas happy and healthy.

Adapting Your Diet to Manage EPI

When it comes to managing EPI, what you eat matters a lot. But fear not, my fellow food lovers, for adapting your diet to accommodate this pesky pancreas problem doesn't mean bidding farewell to delicious meals forever. It's all about making smart choices and finding creative ways to enjoy your favorite foods without aggravating digestive symptoms.

One of the key strategies in EPI management is to focus on foods that are easy to digest and gentle on the pancreas. This means steering clear of greasy, fatty foods that can put undue stress on your digestive system and opting instead for lean proteins, whole grains, fruits, and vegetables. Think grilled chicken breast with steamed broccoli and quinoa, or a colorful salad packed with leafy greens, cherry tomatoes, and avocado.

But don't worry, my fellow foodies, flavor doesn't have to take a back seat in the world of EPI-friendly eating. In fact, there are plenty of herbs, spices, and seasonings that can add a punch of flavor to your meals without causing digestive distress. From zesty lemon juice and fragrant garlic to aromatic basil and fiery chili peppers, the culinary world is your oyster minus the oysters, of course.

Importance of Enzyme Replacement Therapy (ERT)

Now, let's talk about a game-changer in the world of EPI management: Enzyme Replacement Therapy (ERT). Think of ERT as your trusty sidekick in the battle against digestive woes a superhero in capsule form, swooping in to save the day (or rather, your digestion).

ERT works by providing your body with the digestive enzymes it's lacking, helping to break down food more effectively and alleviate symptoms like bloating, gas, and diarrhea. These enzymes usually come in the form of capsules or tablets that you take with meals, allowing them to mingle with your food and work their magic in your digestive tract.

But here's the thing, my savvy reader: timing is everything when it comes to ERT. For optimal results, it's crucial to take your enzyme supplements right before or during meals, ensuring that they're on hand to help with digestion when you need them most. It's like having a team of culinary ninjas in your digestive system, ready to spring into action at a moment's notice.

Key Nutrients and Dietary Considerations

When crafting an EPI-friendly eating plan, it's important to pay attention to more than just your digestive enzymes. You also want to make sure you're getting all the essential nutrients your body needs to thrive. After all, a well-nourished body is better equipped to handle the challenges of EPI and maintain optimal health.

One nutrient that deserves special attention in the world of EPI is fat. Since EPI can impair fat digestion, it's important to choose healthy fats that are easier for your body to process. Think avocado, nuts, seeds, and fatty fish like salmon and trout. These sources of "good" fats not only provide essential nutrients like omega-3 fatty acids but also tend to be easier on the digestive system than their greasy counterparts.

In addition to fat, protein is another key player in the EPI-friendly diet. Protein is essential for muscle repair, immune function, and overall health, so it's important to include plenty of protein-rich foods in your meals. Opt for lean sources of protein like chicken, turkey, fish, tofu, and legumes, and aim to spread your protein intake evenly throughout the day to support optimal digestion and absorption.

Meal Planning Tips for EPI

Now that we've covered the basics of EPI-friendly nutrition, let's talk meal planning. Planning ahead is essential for success in managing EPI, as it allows you to ensure that your meals are balanced, nutritious, and gentle on your digestive system.

One of the keys to successful meal planning with EPI is to focus on small, frequent meals and snacks throughout the day rather than large, heavy meals. This helps to prevent overwhelming your digestive system and can help alleviate symptoms like bloating and discomfort.

When planning your meals, aim to include a balance of protein, carbohydrates, and healthy fats, along with plenty of fruits and vegetables for fiber and essential vitamins and minerals. Experiment with different cooking methods like steaming, baking, and grilling to see which ones work best for you and your digestive system.

Essential Kitchen Tools and Ingredients

Now that we've covered the basics of EPI-friendly eating, let's talk about the tools and ingredients you'll need to stock your kitchen for success.

Having the right equipment and pantry staples on hand can make all the difference when it comes to whipping up delicious, nutritious meals that won't aggravate your digestive symptoms.

Must-Have Kitchen Equipment

First up, let's talk kitchen equipment. While you don't need a fancy, high-tech kitchen to cook EPI-friendly meals, there are a few essential tools that can make your culinary adventures a whole lot easier. Here are a few must-haves for your EPI-friendly kitchen:

- **Food Processor or Blender**: These handy gadgets are perfect for pureeing soups, sauces, and smoothies, making them easier to digest and enjoy.
- **Nonstick Cookware**: Nonstick pans and pots are a godsend for cooking with minimal oil and fat, reducing the risk of digestive discomfort.
- **Steamer Basket**: Steaming is one of the gentlest cooking methods for EPI-friendly foods, preserving their nutrients and flavor while keeping them soft and easy to digest.
- **Sharp Knives**: A good set of sharp knives makes chopping and slicing fruits, vegetables, and meats a breeze, ensuring that your meals are prepared with ease and precision.
- **Digital Kitchen Scale**: Precision is key when it comes to portion control, especially with EPI. A digital kitchen scale can help you measure ingredients accurately and ensure that your meals are balanced and nutritious.

Pantry Staples for EPI-Friendly Cooking

Now let's talk pantry staples the building blocks of any well-stocked kitchen. When it comes to EPI-friendly cooking, it's important to keep your pantry stocked with ingredients that are easy to digest, versatile, and packed with nutrients. Here are a few essentials to keep on hand:

- **Whole Grains**: Opt for whole grains like quinoa, brown rice, oats, and barley, which are rich in fiber and nutrients and easier to digest than refined grains.
- **Legumes**: Beans, lentils, and chickpeas are not only affordable and versatile but also packed with protein, fiber, and essential vitamins and minerals.
- **Healthy Oils**: Choose heart-healthy oils like olive oil, avocado oil, and coconut oil for cooking and dressing salads. These oils are rich in monounsaturated fats and can help support digestive health.
- **Herbs and Spices**: Stock your spice rack with a variety of herbs and spices to add flavor to your meals without adding extra fat or calories. Think basil, oregano, cilantro, cinnamon, ginger, and turmeric the culinary possibilities are endless!
- **Low-FODMAP Foods**: FODMAPs are a group of fermentable carbohydrates that can trigger digestive symptoms in some people, including those with EPI. Opt for low-FODMAP foods like berries, citrus fruits, leafy greens, and lactose-free dairy products to minimize digestive discomfort.

By stocking your kitchen with these essential tools and ingredients, you'll be well-equipped to whip up delicious, nutritious meals that won't aggravate your digestive symptoms. So go ahead, my culinary friend, stock up your pantry, sharpen your knives, and get ready to embark on a delicious journey of EPI-friendly cooking. Your taste buds—and your pancreas will thank you

BEYOND THE BASICS

Welcome to the advanced level of EPI-friendly eating where we dive deeper into the culinary world and explore new horizons of flavor, technique, and dining etiquette. In this chapter, we'll take your EPI management skills to the next level, equipping you with the knowledge and tools you need to navigate a variety of culinary challenges with confidence and ease.

Advanced Cooking Techniques for EPI-Friendly Meals

Let's kick things off with a deep dive into advanced cooking techniques for crafting delicious, digestible meals that won't leave your pancreas in a panic. While the basics of EPI-friendly cooking focus on choosing gentle ingredients and simple preparation methods, advanced techniques allow us to elevate our culinary creations to new heights without sacrificing digestive comfort.

One technique to master is the art of slow cooking. Slow cooking involves cooking food at low temperatures over an extended period, allowing flavors to meld together and proteins to break down into tender, succulent goodness. This gentle cooking method is perfect for EPI-friendly meals, as it helps to break down tough proteins and fibrous vegetables, making them easier to digest while imparting rich, complex flavors to your dishes.

Another advanced technique to explore is sous vide cooking. Sous vide involves cooking food in a vacuum-sealed bag in a temperature-controlled water bath, resulting in perfectly cooked meats, fish, and vegetables every time. This method is ideal for EPI-friendly cooking because it allows you to cook foods gently and evenly without the need for added fats or oils, preserving their natural flavors and nutrients in the process.

In addition to slow cooking and sous vide, consider experimenting with techniques like braising, poaching, and steaming to create tender, flavorful meals that are easy on the digestive system. By mastering these advanced cooking techniques, you'll be able to enjoy a wider variety of foods while keeping your EPI symptoms at bay.

Cooking for Multiple Dietary Restrictions

Now, let's talk about a challenge that many of us face in the kitchen: cooking for multiple dietary restrictions. Whether you're dealing with EPI, food allergies, intolerances, or dietary preferences, accommodating everyone's needs can feel like a daunting task. But fear not, my culinary comrades, for with a little creativity and flexibility, you can create meals that satisfy everyone around the table.

One strategy for cooking for multiple dietary restrictions is to focus on whole, minimally processed foods that are naturally free of common allergens and irritants. Think fruits, vegetables, lean proteins, whole grains, and plant-based fats—the building blocks of a nutritious, inclusive diet. By centering your meals around these wholesome ingredients, you can create dishes that are naturally allergen-friendly and adaptable to a variety of dietary needs.

Another approach is to embrace alternative ingredients and cooking methods to accommodate specific dietary restrictions. For example, if you're cooking for someone with lactose intolerance, you might swap dairy milk for almond milk in recipes or use dairy-free cheese alternatives. Similarly, if you're cooking for someone with gluten sensitivity, you might opt for gluten-free grains like quinoa or rice and use gluten-free flour blends in baking.

International Flavors Made EPI-Friendly

Now, let's embark on a culinary journey around the globe as we explore international flavors made EPI-friendly. One of the joys of food is its ability to transport us to distant lands and immerse us in different cultures through taste and aroma. But for those with EPI, navigating the world of international cuisine can pose some challenges, as many traditional dishes are rich in fats, spices, and hard-to-digest ingredients.

But fear not, my adventurous eaters, for with a little creativity and ingenuity, you can enjoy the bold flavors of international cuisine without sacrificing digestive comfort. One strategy is to focus on dishes that are naturally EPI-friendly or easily adaptable to suit your dietary needs. For example, many Asian cuisines feature light, broth soups, stir-fries, and steamed dishes that are low in fat and gentle on the digestive system. Similarly, Mediterranean cuisine offers a wealth of options like grilled fish, fresh salads, and vegetable-based dishes that are rich in flavor and nutrients.

Another approach is to experiment with alternative ingredients and cooking methods to recreate your favorite international dishes in a way that's EPI-friendly. For example, you might swap heavy cream for coconut milk in Indian curries or use lean cuts of meat in Mexican tacos and fajitas. By getting creative in the kitchen and thinking outside the box, you can enjoy the diverse flavors of global cuisine while keeping your digestive system happy and healthy.

Tips for Dining Out with EPI

Finally, let's talk about everyone's favorite pastime: dining out. Eating out can be a source of joy and relaxation, allowing us to indulge in delicious meals without the hassle of cooking and cleaning. But for those with EPI, dining out can also be a source of anxiety and uncertainty, as navigating restaurant menus and deciphering ingredients can be a challenge.

But fear not, my savvy diners, for with a few simple strategies, you can enjoy dining out with confidence and ease. One tip is to do your homework before heading to the restaurant. Many restaurants now offer online menus with detailed ingredient lists, making it easier to identify EPI-friendly options and plan your meal in advance. If possible, call ahead to speak with the chef or manager about your dietary needs and any special accommodations you may require.

Another strategy is to focus on simple, straightforward dishes that are less likely to contain hidden fats, spices, or hard-to-digest ingredients. Look for grilled or broiled meats, steamed vegetables, and simple salads dressed with olive oil and vinegar. And don't be afraid to ask your server questions about how dishes are prepared and whether any modifications can be made to suit your dietary needs.

BREAKFAST RECIPES

EPI-Friendly Veggie Omelet

Prep Time: 10 mins

Total Time: 15 mins

Servings: 2 servings

Ingredients:

- 4 large eggs
- 1/4 cup chopped bell peppers (any color)
- 1/4 cup diced tomatoes
- 1/4 cup chopped spinach
- 1/4 cup diced mushrooms
- Salt and pepper to taste
- 2 teaspoons olive oil

Directions:

1. In a bowl, beat the eggs until well combined. Season with salt and pepper.
2. Heat 1 teaspoon of olive oil in a non-stick skillet over medium heat.
3. Add the chopped vegetables to the skillet and cook for 2-3 minutes until they begin to soften.
4. Pour the beaten eggs over the vegetables, tilting the skillet to spread them evenly.
5. Cook for 3-4 minutes, or until the eggs are set around the edges.
6. Using a spatula, gently fold the omelet in half and cook for another 1-2 minutes until the eggs are fully cooked.

7. Repeat the process to make the second omelet.
8. Serve hot with a side of whole grain toast or fresh fruit.

Nutrition Facts (per serving):
- Calories: 180
- Protein: 13g
- Fat: 12g
- Carbohydrates: 5g
- Fiber: 2g

EPI-Friendly Banana Oat Pancakes

Prep Time: 5 mins

Total Time: 15 mins

Servings: 2 servings

Ingredients:
- 1 ripe banana, mashed
- 2 large eggs
- 1/2 cup rolled oats
- 1/4 teaspoon cinnamon
- 1/4 teaspoon vanilla extract
- 1/4 cup fresh berries (optional, for topping)
- Maple syrup or honey (optional, for drizzling)

Directions:
1. In a mixing bowl, combine the mashed banana, eggs, rolled oats, cinnamon, and vanilla extract. Mix until well combined.
2. Heat a non-stick skillet or griddle over medium heat and lightly grease with cooking spray or oil.

3. Pour about 1/4 cup of the pancake batter onto the skillet for each pancake.
4. Cook for 2-3 minutes on one side, or until bubbles form on the surface.
5. Flip the pancakes and cook for another 1-2 minutes on the other side, until golden brown and cooked through.
6. Repeat with the remaining batter.
7. Serve the pancakes topped with fresh berries and a drizzle of maple syrup or honey, if desired.

Nutrition Facts (per serving):
- Calories: 220
- Protein: 9g
- Fat: 7g
- Carbohydrates: 32g
- Fiber: 4g

EPI-Friendly Greek Yogurt Parfait

Prep Time: 5 mins

Total Time: 5 mins

Servings: 1 serving

Ingredients:
- 1/2 cup plain Greek yogurt
- 1/4 cup granola (choose a low-sugar option)
- 1/4 cup mixed berries (such as strawberries, blueberries, raspberries)
- 1 tablespoon honey or maple syrup (optional)

Directions:

1. In a glass or bowl, layer the Greek yogurt, granola, and mixed berries.
2. Drizzle with honey or maple syrup, if desired.
3. Serve immediately and enjoy!

Nutrition Facts (per serving):
- Calories: 250
- Protein: 18g
- Fat: 6g
- Carbohydrates: 33g
- Fiber: 5g

EPI-Friendly Avocado Toast

Prep Time: 5 mins

Total Time: 10 mins

Servings: 1 serving

Ingredients:
- 1 slice whole grain bread, toasted
- 1/2 ripe avocado
- 1/4 teaspoon red pepper flakes (optional)
- 1 teaspoon lemon juice
- Salt and pepper to taste

Directions:
1. Mash the avocado in a small bowl with a fork until smooth.
2. Stir in the lemon juice, red pepper flakes (if using), salt, and pepper.
3. Spread the mashed avocado mixture evenly onto the toasted bread.

4. Serve immediately and enjoy!

Nutrition Facts (per serving):
- Calories: 180
- Protein: 4g
- Fat: 10g
- Carbohydrates: 20g
- Fiber: 6g

EPI-Friendly Berry Smoothie Bowl

Prep Time: 5 mins

Total Time: 5 mins

Servings: 1 serving

Ingredients:
- 1/2 cup frozen mixed berries (such as strawberries, blueberries, raspberries)
- 1/2 ripe banana
- 1/2 cup plain Greek yogurt
- 1/4 cup almond milk (or any milk of your choice)
- 1 tablespoon chia seeds
- 1 tablespoon honey or maple syrup (optional)
- Toppings: sliced banana, fresh berries, granola, shredded coconut

Directions:
1. In a blender, combine the frozen berries, banana, Greek yogurt, almond milk, chia seeds, and honey or maple syrup (if using).
2. Blend until smooth and creamy, adding more almond milk if needed to reach your desired consistency.

3. Pour the smoothie into a bowl and top with sliced banana, fresh berries, granola, and shredded coconut.
4. Serve immediately and enjoy!

Nutrition Facts (per serving):
- Calories: 280
- Protein: 15g
- Fat: 8g
- Carbohydrates: 40g
- Fiber: 9g

Soothing Banana Porridge

Prep Time: 5 mins

Total Time: 10 mins

Servings: 2

Ingredients:
- 1 ripe banana, mashed
- 1 cup rolled oats
- 2 cups water or almond milk
- 1/2 teaspoon cinnamon
- Pinch of salt
- 1 tablespoon honey or maple syrup (optional)
- Fresh berries or sliced banana for topping

Directions:
1. In a saucepan, combine the mashed banana, rolled oats, water or almond milk, cinnamon, and salt.

2. Bring to a boil over medium-high heat, then reduce the heat to low and simmer for 5-7 minutes, stirring occasionally, until the oats are cooked and the mixture has thickened.
3. Remove from heat and stir in the honey or maple syrup, if using.
4. Divide the porridge into bowls and top with fresh berries or sliced banana.
5. Serve warm and enjoy!

Nutrition Facts (per serving):
- Calories: 210
- Protein: 5g
- Fat: 2g
- Carbohydrates: 44g
- Fiber: 6g

Savory Spinach and Mushroom Scramble

Prep Time: 5 mins

Total Time: 10 mins

Servings: 2

Ingredients:
- 4 large eggs
- 1 cup chopped spinach
- 1/2 cup sliced mushrooms
- 1/4 cup diced onion
- 1 tablespoon olive oil
- Salt and pepper to taste
- Fresh herbs (such as parsley or chives) for garnish

Directions:
1. In a bowl, whisk the eggs until well combined. Season with salt and pepper.
2. Heat the olive oil in a skillet over medium heat.
3. Add the diced onion and cook for 2-3 minutes until softened.
4. Add the sliced mushrooms to the skillet and cook for another 2-3 minutes until they begin to brown.
5. Add the chopped spinach to the skillet and cook for 1-2 minutes until wilted.
6. Pour the beaten eggs into the skillet and cook, stirring gently, until the eggs are scrambled and cooked to your desired consistency.
7. Divide the scramble onto plates and garnish with fresh herbs.
8. Serve hot and enjoy!

Nutrition Facts (per serving):
- Calories: 180
- Protein: 12g
- Fat: 13g
- Carbohydrates: 5g
- Fiber: 2g

Ginger Turmeric Smoothie

Prep Time: 5 mins

Total Time: 5 mins

Servings: 2

Ingredients:
- 1 cup frozen mango chunks

- 1 ripe banana
- 1 cup coconut water or almond milk
- 1/2 teaspoon grated fresh ginger
- 1/2 teaspoon ground turmeric
- 1 tablespoon honey or maple syrup (optional)
- Pinch of black pepper (to activate turmeric)

Directions:

1. In a blender, combine the frozen mango chunks, banana, coconut water or almond milk, grated ginger, ground turmeric, honey or maple syrup (if using), and black pepper.
2. Blend until smooth and creamy.
3. Pour into glasses and serve immediately.
4. Enjoy the refreshing and anti-inflammatory benefits of this vibrant smoothie!

Nutrition Facts (per serving):

- Calories: 150
- Protein: 2g
- Fat: 1g
- Carbohydrates: 37g
- Fiber: 4g

Quinoa Breakfast Bowl

Prep Time: 5 mins

Total Time: 20 mins

Servings: 2

Ingredients:

- 1/2 cup quinoa, rinsed

- 1 cup water or almond milk
- 1/2 teaspoon cinnamon
- 1 tablespoon honey or maple syrup (optional)
- 1/4 cup chopped nuts (such as almonds, walnuts, or pecans)
- 1/4 cup dried fruit (such as raisins, cranberries, or apricots)
- Fresh berries or sliced banana for topping

Directions:
1. In a saucepan, combine the quinoa, water or almond milk, cinnamon, and honey or maple syrup (if using).
2. Bring to a boil over medium-high heat, then reduce the heat to low and simmer for 15-20 minutes, or until the quinoa is cooked and the liquid has been absorbed.
3. Fluff the quinoa with a fork and divide it into bowls.
4. Top with chopped nuts, dried fruit, and fresh berries or sliced banana.
5. Serve warm and enjoy this hearty and nutritious breakfast bowl!

Nutrition Facts (per serving):
- Calories: 280
- Protein: 9g
- Fat: 8g
- Carbohydrates: 47g
- Fiber: 6g

Energizing Chia Seed Pudding

Prep Time: 5 mins

Total Time: 2 hours 5 mins (includes chilling time)

Servings: 2

Ingredients:
- 1/4 cup chia seeds
- 1 cup almond milk or coconut milk
- 1 tablespoon honey or maple syrup
- 1/2 teaspoon vanilla extract
- Fresh fruit for topping (such as berries, sliced banana, or kiwi)

Directions:
1. In a mixing bowl, combine the chia seeds, almond milk or coconut milk, honey or maple syrup, and vanilla extract.
2. Whisk together until well combined.
3. Cover the bowl and refrigerate for at least 2 hours, or preferably overnight, to allow the chia seeds to thicken and absorb the liquid.
4. Stir the pudding well before serving to ensure a smooth consistency.
5. Divide the chia seed pudding into serving glasses or bowls.
6. Top with fresh fruit and enjoy this nutrient-rich and energizing breakfast treat!

Nutrition Facts (per serving):
- Calories: 150
- Protein: 4g
- Fat: 7g
- Carbohydrates: 18g
- Fiber: 9g

Hearty Quinoa Breakfast Bowl

Prep Time: 5 mins

Total Time: 20 mins

Servings: 2

Ingredients:

- 1/2 cup quinoa, rinsed
- 1 cup water or almond milk
- 1/2 teaspoon cinnamon
- 1 tablespoon honey or maple syrup (optional)
- 1/4 cup chopped nuts (such as almonds, walnuts, or pecans)
- 1/4 cup dried fruit (such as raisins, cranberries, or apricots)
- Fresh berries or sliced banana for topping

Directions:

1. In a saucepan, combine the quinoa, water or almond milk, cinnamon, and honey or maple syrup (if using).
2. Bring to a boil over medium-high heat, then reduce the heat to low and simmer for 15-20 minutes, or until the quinoa is cooked and the liquid has been absorbed.
3. Fluff the quinoa with a fork and divide it into bowls.
4. Top with chopped nuts, dried fruit, and fresh berries or sliced banana.
5. Serve warm and enjoy this hearty and nutritious breakfast bowl!

Nutrition Facts (per serving):

- Calories: 280
- Protein: 9g
- Fat: 8g
- Carbohydrates: 47g

- Fiber: 6g

Energizing Chia Seed Pudding

Prep Time: 5 mins

Total Time: 2 hours 5 mins (includes chilling time)

Servings: 2

Ingredients:
- 1/4 cup chia seeds
- 1 cup almond milk or coconut milk
- 1 tablespoon honey or maple syrup
- 1/2 teaspoon vanilla extract
- Fresh fruit for topping (such as berries, sliced banana, or kiwi)

Directions:
1. In a mixing bowl, combine the chia seeds, almond milk or coconut milk, honey or maple syrup, and vanilla extract.
2. Whisk together until well combined.
3. Cover the bowl and refrigerate for at least 2 hours, or preferably overnight, to allow the chia seeds to thicken and absorb the liquid.
4. Stir the pudding well before serving to ensure a smooth consistency.
5. Divide the chia seed pudding into serving glasses or bowls.
6. Top with fresh fruit and enjoy this nutrient-rich and energizing breakfast treat!

Nutrition Facts (per serving):
- Calories: 150
- Protein: 4g

- Fat: 7g
- Carbohydrates: 18g
- Fiber: 9g

Zesty Spinach and Egg Muffins

Prep Time: 10 mins

Total Time: 25 mins

Servings: 4

Ingredients:
- 4 large eggs
- 1 cup chopped spinach
- 1/4 cup diced tomatoes
- 1/4 cup diced bell peppers
- 1/4 cup shredded cheddar cheese
- Salt and pepper to taste

Directions:
1. Preheat the oven to 350°F (175°C). Grease a muffin tin with cooking spray or line with paper liners.
2. In a mixing bowl, whisk the eggs until well beaten. Season with salt and pepper.
3. Stir in the chopped spinach, diced tomatoes, diced bell peppers, and shredded cheddar cheese.
4. Divide the egg mixture evenly among the muffin cups.
5. Bake for 15-20 minutes, or until the egg muffins are set and lightly golden on top.
6. Allow the muffins to cool slightly before serving.

7. Enjoy these flavorful and protein-packed egg muffins as a satisfying breakfast option!

Nutrition Facts (per serving - 2 muffins):
- Calories: 180
- Protein: 12g
- Fat: 11g
- Carbohydrates: 6g
- Fiber: 2g

Soothing Banana Porridge

Prep Time: 5 mins

Total Time: 10 mins

Servings: 2

Ingredients:
- 1 ripe banana, mashed
- 1 cup rolled oats
- 2 cups water or almond milk
- 1/2 teaspoon cinnamon
- Pinch of salt
- 1 tablespoon honey or maple syrup (optional)
- Fresh berries or sliced banana for topping

Directions:
1. In a saucepan, combine the mashed banana, rolled oats, water or almond milk, cinnamon, and salt.
2. Bring to a boil over medium-high heat, then reduce the heat to low and simmer for 5-7 minutes, stirring occasionally, until the oats are cooked and the mixture has thickened.

3. Remove from heat and stir in the honey or maple syrup, if using.
4. Divide the porridge into bowls and top with fresh berries or sliced banana.
5. Serve warm and enjoy!

Nutrition Facts (per serving):
- Calories: 210
- Protein: 5g
- Fat: 2g
- Carbohydrates: 44g
- Fiber: 6g

Savory Sweet Potato Hash

Prep Time: 10 mins

Total Time: 25 mins

Servings: 2

Ingredients:
- 1 large sweet potato, peeled and diced
- 1/2 onion, diced
- 1 bell pepper, diced
- 2 cloves garlic, minced
- 2 tablespoons olive oil
- Salt and pepper to taste
- 2 eggs (optional)
- Fresh parsley or cilantro for garnish

Directions:
1. Heat olive oil in a large skillet over medium heat.

2. Add diced sweet potato to the skillet and cook for about 5 minutes, stirring occasionally, until they begin to soften.
3. Add diced onion, bell pepper, and minced garlic to the skillet. Cook for an additional 7-8 minutes, or until the vegetables are tender and slightly caramelized.
4. Season with salt and pepper to taste.
5. If desired, create wells in the hash and crack eggs into each well. Cover the skillet and cook for 3-4 minutes, or until the eggs are cooked to your liking.
6. Garnish with fresh parsley or cilantro before serving.
7. Serve hot and enjoy this satisfying and nutrient-rich breakfast!

Nutrition Facts (per serving without eggs):
- Calories: 250
- Protein: 4g
- Fat: 14g
- Carbohydrates: 29g
- Fiber: 5g

Protein-Packed Scrambled Tofu

Prep Time: 10 mins

Total Time: 15 mins

Servings: 2

Ingredients:
- 1 block (14 oz) firm tofu, drained and crumbled
- 1 tablespoon olive oil
- 1/2 onion, diced
- 1 bell pepper, diced

- 1 cup spinach, chopped
- 2 tablespoons nutritional yeast
- 1/2 teaspoon turmeric powder
- Salt and pepper to taste
- Fresh parsley for garnish

Directions:
1. Heat olive oil in a skillet over medium heat.
2. Add diced onion and bell pepper to the skillet. Cook for 3-4 minutes until softened.
3. Add crumbled tofu to the skillet along with nutritional yeast, turmeric powder, salt, and pepper. Stir well to combine.
4. Cook for another 5-7 minutes, stirring occasionally, until the tofu is heated through and slightly browned.
5. Add chopped spinach to the skillet and cook for an additional 2 minutes until wilted.
6. Garnish with fresh parsley before serving.
7. Enjoy this protein-packed and flavorful breakfast option!

Nutrition Facts (per serving):
- Calories: 220
- Protein: 18g
- Fat: 13g
- Carbohydrates: 10g
- Fiber: 3g

Oatmeal Breakfast Cookies

Prep Time: 10 mins

Total Time: 20 mins

Servings: 8 cookies

Ingredients:

- 1 ripe banana, mashed
- 1/4 cup almond butter
- 1/4 cup honey or maple syrup
- 1 cup rolled oats
- 1/4 cup chopped nuts (such as almonds, walnuts, or pecans)
- 1/4 cup dried fruit (such as raisins, cranberries, or apricots)
- 1/2 teaspoon cinnamon
- Pinch of salt

Directions:

1. Preheat the oven to 350°F (175°C). Line a baking sheet with parchment paper.
2. In a mixing bowl, combine the mashed banana, almond butter, and honey or maple syrup.
3. Stir in the rolled oats, chopped nuts, dried fruit, cinnamon, and salt until well combined.
4. Scoop spoonfuls of the dough onto the prepared baking sheet and flatten slightly with the back of a spoon.
5. Bake for 12-15 minutes, or until the cookies are golden brown around the edges.
6. Remove from the oven and let cool on the baking sheet for 5 minutes before transferring to a wire rack to cool completely.

7. Enjoy these wholesome oatmeal breakfast cookies as a convenient and satisfying grab-and-go option!

Nutrition Facts (per serving - 1 cookie):
- Calories: 150
- Protein: 4g
- Fat: 8g
- Carbohydrates: 18g
- Fiber: 2g

Egg and Veggie Breakfast Burrito

Prep Time: 10 mins

Total Time: 15 mins

Servings: 2

Ingredients:
- 4 large eggs
- 1/2 bell pepper, diced
- 1/2 onion, diced
- 1/2 cup black beans, drained and rinsed
- 1/4 cup shredded cheddar cheese
- 2 whole grain tortillas
- Salt and pepper to taste
- Salsa and avocado slices for serving (optional)

Directions:
1. In a skillet, heat olive oil over medium heat. Add diced bell pepper and onion, sauté until softened, about 3-4 minutes.

2. Crack eggs into the skillet, scramble until cooked through, then mix in black beans and shredded cheddar cheese. Season with salt and pepper to taste.
3. Warm tortillas in a separate skillet or microwave.
4. Divide the egg and veggie mixture evenly between the tortillas, then fold into burritos.
5. Serve with salsa and avocado slices on the side, if desired.
6. Enjoy this hearty and satisfying breakfast burrito!

Nutrition Facts (per serving):
- Calories: 350
- Protein: 20g
- Fat: 15g
- Carbohydrates: 30g
- Fiber: 8g

Creamy Coconut Chia Pudding

Prep Time: 5 mins

Total Time: 2 hours 5 mins (includes chilling time)

Servings: 2

Ingredients:
- 1/4 cup chia seeds
- 1 cup coconut milk
- 1 tablespoon honey or maple syrup
- 1/2 teaspoon vanilla extract
- Fresh fruit for topping (such as berries, sliced banana, or mango)

Directions:

1. In a mixing bowl, combine the chia seeds, coconut milk, honey or maple syrup, and vanilla extract.
2. Whisk together until well combined.
3. Cover the bowl and refrigerate for at least 2 hours, or preferably overnight, to allow the chia seeds to thicken and absorb the liquid.
4. Stir the pudding well before serving to ensure a smooth consistency.
5. Divide the chia seed pudding into serving glasses or bowls.
6. Top with fresh fruit and enjoy this creamy and satisfying breakfast treat!

Nutrition Facts (per serving):
- Calories: 230
- Protein: 5g
- Fat: 17g
- Carbohydrates: 17g
- Fiber: 9g

Berry Banana Smoothie Bowl

Prep Time: 5 mins

Total Time: 5 mins

Servings: 2

Ingredients:
- 1 ripe banana
- 1 cup frozen mixed berries (such as strawberries, blueberries, raspberries)
- 1/2 cup plain Greek yogurt

- 1/4 cup almond milk or coconut water
- 1 tablespoon chia seeds
- 1 tablespoon honey or maple syrup (optional)
- Toppings: sliced banana, fresh berries, granola, shredded coconut

Directions:

1. In a blender, combine the ripe banana, frozen mixed berries, Greek yogurt, almond milk or coconut water, chia seeds, and honey or maple syrup (if using).
2. Blend until smooth and creamy, adding more almond milk or coconut water if needed to reach your desired consistency.
3. Pour the smoothie into bowls.
4. Top with sliced banana, fresh berries, granola, and shredded coconut.
5. Serve immediately and enjoy this refreshing and nutritious smoothie bowl!

Nutrition Facts (per serving):

- Calories: 250
- Protein: 9g
- Fat: 7g
- Carbohydrates: 40g
- Fiber: 9g

SNACKS RECIPES

Nutty Energy Bites

Prep Time: 15 mins

Total Time: 15 mins

Servings: 12 bites

Ingredients:
- 1 cup rolled oats
- 1/2 cup creamy almond butter
- 1/4 cup honey or maple syrup
- 1/4 cup chopped nuts (such as almonds, walnuts, or cashews)
- 1/4 cup dried fruit (such as raisins, cranberries, or apricots), chopped
- 1 tablespoon chia seeds
- 1/2 teaspoon vanilla extract
- Pinch of salt

Directions:
1. In a large mixing bowl, combine rolled oats, almond butter, honey or maple syrup, chopped nuts, dried fruit, chia seeds, vanilla extract, and a pinch of salt.
2. Stir until well combined and the mixture holds together.
3. Using your hands, roll the mixture into small balls, about 1 inch in diameter.
4. Place the energy bites on a baking sheet lined with parchment paper.
5. Refrigerate for at least 30 minutes to firm up.

6. Once firm, transfer the energy bites to an airtight container and store in the refrigerator for up to 1 week.
7. Enjoy these nutritious and satisfying energy bites as a quick and convenient snack!

Nutrition Facts (per serving - 1 bite):
- Calories: 120
- Protein: 3g
- Fat: 6g
- Carbohydrates: 14g
- Fiber: 2g

Avocado Toast with Tomato and Basil

Prep Time: 5 mins

Total Time: 10 mins

Servings: 2

Ingredients:
- 2 slices whole grain bread, toasted
- 1 ripe avocado, mashed
- 1 tomato, sliced
- Fresh basil leaves
- Salt and pepper to taste
- Optional toppings: red pepper flakes, balsamic glaze

Directions:
1. Spread the mashed avocado evenly onto the toasted whole grain bread slices.
2. Top each slice with tomato slices and fresh basil leaves.
3. Season with salt and pepper to taste.

4. For added flavor, sprinkle with red pepper flakes and drizzle with balsamic glaze, if desired.
5. Serve immediately and enjoy this simple and delicious avocado toast!

Nutrition Facts (per serving):
- Calories: 180
- Protein: 5g
- Fat: 10g
- Carbohydrates: 20g
- Fiber: 8g

Greek Yogurt Parfait

Prep Time: 5 mins

Total Time: 5 mins

Servings: 1

Ingredients:
- 1/2 cup plain Greek yogurt
- 1/4 cup granola
- 1/4 cup mixed berries (such as strawberries, blueberries, raspberries)
- 1 tablespoon honey or maple syrup (optional)

Directions:
1. In a serving glass or bowl, layer the plain Greek yogurt, granola, and mixed berries.
2. Drizzle with honey or maple syrup, if using.
3. Repeat the layers until the glass or bowl is full.

4. Serve immediately and enjoy this creamy and refreshing Greek yogurt parfait!

Nutrition Facts (per serving):
- Calories: 250
- Protein: 15g
- Fat: 6g
- Carbohydrates: 35g
- Fiber: 5g

Hummus and Veggie Stuffed Pita Pockets

Prep Time: 10 mins

Total Time: 10 mins

Servings: 2

Ingredients:
- 2 whole grain pita pockets
- 1/2 cup hummus
- 1/2 cucumber, thinly sliced
- 1/2 bell pepper, thinly sliced
- 1/4 cup shredded carrots
- Handful of spinach leaves

Directions:
1. Warm the whole grain pita pockets in the microwave or toaster oven until slightly soft and pliable.
2. Carefully cut open each pita pocket to create a pocket for filling.
3. Spread a generous amount of hummus inside each pita pocket.

4. Stuff each pocket with cucumber slices, bell pepper slices, shredded carrots, and spinach leaves.
5. Serve immediately and enjoy these delicious and nutritious stuffed pita pockets as a satisfying snack!

Nutrition Facts (per serving):
- Calories: 280
- Protein: 10g
- Fat: 8g
- Carbohydrates: 45g
- Fiber: 8g

Vegetable Sushi Rolls

Prep Time: 20 mins

Total Time: 20 mins

Servings: 2

Ingredients:
- 2 nori seaweed sheets
- 1 cup cooked sushi rice
- 1/2 cucumber, julienned
- 1/2 carrot, julienned
- 1/2 avocado, sliced
- 2 tablespoons rice vinegar
- 1 tablespoon soy sauce or tamari
- Pickled ginger and wasabi for serving (optional)

Directions:
1. Place a nori seaweed sheet on a bamboo sushi mat or clean kitchen towel.

2. Spread a thin layer of cooked sushi rice evenly over the nori sheet, leaving about 1 inch of space at the top.
3. Arrange cucumber, carrot, and avocado slices in a row along the bottom edge of the rice.
4. Using the sushi mat or towel, tightly roll up the nori sheet, pressing gently to seal the roll.
5. Repeat with the remaining ingredients to make the second sushi roll.
6. Use a sharp knife to slice each roll into bite-sized pieces.
7. Serve with soy sauce or tamari, pickled ginger, and wasabi on the side, if desired.
8. Enjoy these homemade vegetable sushi rolls as a healthy and flavorful snack!

Nutrition Facts (per serving - 1 roll):
- Calories: 220
- Protein: 5g
- Fat: 5g
- Carbohydrates: 40g
- Fiber: 5g

Crunchy Chickpea Snack

Prep Time: 5 mins

Total Time: 25 mins

Servings: 2

Ingredients:
- 1 can (15 oz) chickpeas, drained and rinsed
- 1 tablespoon olive oil

- 1 teaspoon paprika
- 1/2 teaspoon garlic powder
- 1/2 teaspoon cumin
- Salt and pepper to taste

Directions:
1. Preheat the oven to 400°F (200°C). Line a baking sheet with parchment paper.
2. Pat the chickpeas dry with a clean kitchen towel or paper towel.
3. In a mixing bowl, toss the chickpeas with olive oil, paprika, garlic powder, cumin, salt, and pepper until evenly coated.
4. Spread the chickpeas in a single layer on the prepared baking sheet.
5. Bake for 20-25 minutes, or until crispy and golden brown, stirring halfway through.
6. Remove from the oven and let cool before serving.
7. Enjoy these crunchy chickpeas as a satisfying and flavorful snack!

Nutrition Facts (per serving):
- Calories: 150
- Protein: 6g
- Fat: 7g
- Carbohydrates: 18g
- Fiber: 5g

Apple and Peanut Butter Rice Cakes

Prep Time: 5 mins

Total Time: 5 mins

Servings: 2

Ingredients:

- 2 rice cakes (whole grain or gluten-free)
- 2 tablespoons natural peanut butter
- 1 small apple, thinly sliced
- Cinnamon for sprinkling (optional)

Directions:

1. Spread a tablespoon of peanut butter onto each rice cake.
2. Arrange thinly sliced apple on top of the peanut butter.
3. Sprinkle with cinnamon, if desired.
4. Serve immediately and enjoy this simple and satisfying snack!

Nutrition Facts (per serving):

- Calories: 200
- Protein: 5g
- Fat: 10g
- Carbohydrates: 25g
- Fiber: 5g

Vegetable Crudité with Hummus

Prep Time: 10 mins

Total Time: 10 mins

Servings: 2

Ingredients:

- Assorted raw vegetables (such as baby carrots, cucumber sticks, bell pepper strips, cherry tomatoes)

- 1/2 cup hummus

Directions:
1. Wash and prepare the raw vegetables by cutting them into sticks or bite-sized pieces.
2. Arrange the vegetable crudité on a serving platter.
3. Serve with hummus for dipping.
4. Enjoy this colorful and nutritious snack!

Nutrition Facts (per serving):
- Calories: 150
- Protein: 6g
- Fat: 7g
- Carbohydrates: 20g
- Fiber: 7g

Quinoa and Black Bean Salad Cups

Prep Time: 10 mins

Total Time: 10 mins

Servings: 2

Ingredients:
- 1 cup cooked quinoa
- 1/2 cup black beans, drained and rinsed
- 1/4 cup diced bell pepper
- 1/4 cup diced cucumber
- 1/4 cup cherry tomatoes, halved
- 2 tablespoons chopped fresh cilantro
- Juice of 1 lime
- Salt and pepper to taste

Directions:
1. In a mixing bowl, combine cooked quinoa, black beans, diced bell pepper, diced cucumber, cherry tomatoes, chopped fresh cilantro, lime juice, salt, and pepper.
2. Stir until well combined.
3. Spoon the quinoa and black bean salad into small cups or bowls for serving.
4. Enjoy this refreshing and protein-packed snack!

Nutrition Facts (per serving):
- Calories: 200
- Protein: 8g
- Fat: 2g
- Carbohydrates: 38g
- Fiber: 7g

Banana Almond Butter Bites

Prep Time: 5 mins

Total Time: 5 mins

Servings: 2

Ingredients:
- 1 large banana, sliced
- 2 tablespoons almond butter
- 2 tablespoons granola

Directions:
1. Spread almond butter onto banana slices.
2. Sprinkle granola on top of almond butter.

3. Serve immediately and enjoy these delicious and satisfying bites!

Nutrition Facts (per serving):
- Calories: 180
- Protein: 4g
- Fat: 9g
- Carbohydrates: 22g
- Fiber: 3g

Zesty Cucumber Hummus Cups

Prep Time: 10 mins

Total Time: 10 mins

Servings: 2

Ingredients:
- 1 cucumber
- 1/2 cup hummus
- Cherry tomatoes, sliced
- Black olives, sliced
- Fresh parsley, chopped

Directions:
1. Wash the cucumber and cut it into thick slices, about 1 inch thick.
2. Use a melon baller or small spoon to scoop out some of the seeds from the center of each cucumber slice, creating a cup-like shape.
3. Fill each cucumber cup with a spoonful of hummus.

4. Top with sliced cherry tomatoes, black olives, and chopped parsley.
5. Serve immediately and enjoy these refreshing and flavorful hummus cups!

Nutrition Facts (per serving):
- Calories: 100
- Protein: 5g
- Fat: 5g
- Carbohydrates: 10g
- Fiber: 4g

Crispy Baked Kale Chips

Prep Time: 10 mins

Total Time: 25 mins

Servings: 2

Ingredients:
- 1 bunch kale
- 1 tablespoon olive oil
- Salt and pepper to taste
- Optional: nutritional yeast, garlic powder, chili flakes

Directions:
1. Preheat the oven to 300°F (150°C). Line a baking sheet with parchment paper.
2. Wash the kale leaves and pat them dry with a clean kitchen towel or paper towel.
3. Remove the tough stems from the kale leaves and tear the leaves into bite-sized pieces.

4. In a large mixing bowl, toss the kale pieces with olive oil, salt, pepper, and any optional seasonings of your choice.
5. Spread the seasoned kale pieces in a single layer on the prepared baking sheet.
6. Bake for 20-25 minutes, or until the kale chips are crispy and slightly golden brown, stirring halfway through.
7. Remove from the oven and let cool before serving.
8. Enjoy these crispy kale chips as a nutritious and satisfying snack!

Nutrition Facts (per serving):
- Calories: 80
- Protein: 5g
- Fat: 4g
- Carbohydrates: 10g
- Fiber: 3g

Sweet Potato Toasts with Almond Butter

Prep Time: 5 mins

Total Time: 15 mins

Servings: 2

Ingredients:
- 1 large sweet potato
- 2 tablespoons almond butter
- Optional toppings: sliced banana, chia seeds, cinnamon

Directions:
1. Wash the sweet potato and slice it lengthwise into thin slices, about 1/4 inch thick.

2. Toast the sweet potato slices in a toaster or toaster oven until they are cooked through and slightly crispy.
3. Spread a tablespoon of almond butter onto each sweet potato slice.
4. Top with sliced banana, chia seeds, and a sprinkle of cinnamon, if desired.
5. Serve immediately and enjoy these delicious and nutritious sweet potato toasts!

Nutrition Facts (per serving):
- Calories: 150
- Protein: 3g
- Fat: 8g
- Carbohydrates: 18g
- Fiber: 3g

Mango Salsa with Whole Grain Crackers

Prep Time: 10 mins

Total Time: 10 mins

Servings: 2

Ingredients:
- 1 ripe mango, diced
- 1/4 cup red onion, finely chopped
- 1/4 cup fresh cilantro, chopped
- 1 jalapeño pepper, seeded and finely chopped
- Juice of 1 lime
- Salt and pepper to taste
- Whole grain crackers for serving

Directions:
1. In a mixing bowl, combine diced mango, chopped red onion, chopped cilantro, chopped jalapeño pepper, lime juice, salt, and pepper. Stir until well combined.
2. Taste and adjust seasoning, if needed.
3. Serve the mango salsa with whole grain crackers for dipping.
4. Enjoy this vibrant and flavorful salsa as a delicious and wholesome snack!

Nutrition Facts (per serving):
- Calories: 120
- Protein: 2g
- Fat: 1g
- Carbohydrates: 30g
- Fiber: 4g

Quinoa-Stuffed Bell Pepper

Prep Time: 15 mins

Total Time: 45 mins

Servings: 2

Ingredients:
- 2 large bell peppers (any color), halved and seeds removed
- 1/2 cup cooked quinoa
- 1/2 cup cooked black beans, drained and rinsed
- 1/4 cup corn kernels
- 1/4 cup diced tomatoes
- 1/4 cup diced red onion
- 1/4 cup diced avocado

- 1/4 cup chopped fresh cilantro
- Juice of 1 lime
- Salt and pepper to taste
- Optional: shredded cheese, salsa

Directions:

1. Preheat the oven to 375°F (190°C). Place the halved bell peppers on a baking sheet.
2. In a mixing bowl, combine cooked quinoa, black beans, corn kernels, diced tomatoes, diced red onion, diced avocado, chopped cilantro, lime juice, salt, and pepper. Stir until well combined.
3. Spoon the quinoa mixture into each bell pepper half, pressing down gently to fill.
4. If desired, sprinkle shredded cheese on top of each stuffed bell pepper.
5. Bake for 25-30 minutes, or until the bell peppers are tender and the filling is heated through.
6. Remove from the oven and let cool slightly before serving.
7. Serve with salsa on the side, if desired.
8. Enjoy these flavorful and nutritious quinoa-stuffed bell peppers as a satisfying snack or light meal!

Nutrition Facts (per serving):

- Calories: 250
- Protein: 9g
- Fat: 6g
- Carbohydrates: 40g

- Fiber: 9g

Nutty Banana Oat Bars

Prep Time: 10 mins

Total Time: 30 mins

Servings: 8 bars

Ingredients:

- 2 ripe bananas, mashed
- 1 cup rolled oats
- 1/4 cup almond butter
- 1/4 cup chopped nuts (such as almonds, walnuts, or cashews)
- 1/4 cup dried fruit (such as raisins, cranberries, or apricots), chopped
- 1 tablespoon honey or maple syrup
- 1 teaspoon cinnamon
- Pinch of salt

Directions:

1. Preheat the oven to 350°F (175°C). Grease a baking dish or line it with parchment paper.
2. In a mixing bowl, combine mashed bananas, rolled oats, almond butter, chopped nuts, dried fruit, honey or maple syrup, cinnamon, and a pinch of salt. Stir until well combined.
3. Press the mixture evenly into the prepared baking dish.
4. Bake for 20-25 minutes, or until the bars are golden brown and firm to the touch.
5. Remove from the oven and let cool before slicing into bars.
6. Once cooled, cut into bars and store in an airtight container.

7. Enjoy these nutty banana oat bars as a wholesome and energizing snack!

Nutrition Facts (per serving):
- Calories: 150
- Protein: 4g
- Fat: 7g
- Carbohydrates: 20g
- Fiber: 3g

Roasted Chickpea Trail Mix

Prep Time: 10 mins

Total Time: 40 mins

Servings: 4

Ingredients:
- 1 can (15 oz) chickpeas, drained and rinsed
- 1 tablespoon olive oil
- 1 teaspoon ground cumin
- 1 teaspoon chili powder
- 1/2 teaspoon garlic powder
- 1/2 teaspoon paprika
- 1/4 teaspoon salt
- 1/4 cup dried cranberries
- 1/4 cup roasted almonds
- 1/4 cup pumpkin seeds
- 1/4 cup dark chocolate chips

Directions:

1. Preheat the oven to 400°F (200°C). Line a baking sheet with parchment paper.
2. Pat the chickpeas dry with a clean kitchen towel or paper towel.
3. In a mixing bowl, toss the chickpeas with olive oil, ground cumin, chili powder, garlic powder, paprika, and salt until evenly coated.
4. Spread the seasoned chickpeas in a single layer on the prepared baking sheet.
5. Roast for 30-35 minutes, stirring halfway through, until the chickpeas are crispy and golden brown.
6. Remove from the oven and let cool completely.
7. Once cooled, transfer the roasted chickpeas to a mixing bowl and add dried cranberries, roasted almonds, pumpkin seeds, and dark chocolate chips. Toss to combine.
8. Store the roasted chickpea trail mix in an airtight container for up to 1 week.
9. Enjoy this crunchy and flavorful trail mix as a satisfying snack on the go!

Nutrition Facts (per serving):
- Calories: 250
- Protein: 8g
- Fat: 10g
- Carbohydrates: 30g
- Fiber: 6g

Greek Yogurt Berry Parfait

Prep Time: 5 mins

Total Time: 5 mins

Servings: 2

Ingredients:

- 1 cup plain Greek yogurt
- 1/2 cup mixed berries (such as strawberries, blueberries, raspberries)
- 1/4 cup granola
- 1 tablespoon honey or maple syrup (optional)

Directions:

1. In a serving glass or bowl, layer the plain Greek yogurt, mixed berries, and granola.
2. Drizzle with honey or maple syrup, if using.
3. Repeat the layers until the glass or bowl is full.
4. Serve immediately and enjoy this creamy and nutritious Greek yogurt berry parfait!

Nutrition Facts (per serving):

- Calories: 180
- Protein: 15g
- Fat: 3g
- Carbohydrates: 30g
- Fiber: 3g

Stuffed Celery Sticks

Prep Time: 10 mins

Total Time: 10 mins

Servings: 2

Ingredients:
- 4 celery stalks, washed and trimmed
- 1/4 cup hummus
- 1/4 cup sliced almonds
- 1/4 cup dried cranberries

Directions:
1. Cut the celery stalks into halves or thirds, depending on their size.
2. Fill each celery stick with hummus.
3. Top with sliced almonds and dried cranberries.
4. Serve immediately and enjoy these crunchy and flavorful stuffed celery sticks!

Nutrition Facts (per serving):
- Calories: 120
- Protein: 4g
- Fat: 7g
- Carbohydrates: 12g
- Fiber: 4g

Turkey and Avocado Roll-Ups

Prep Time: 10 mins

Total Time: 10 mins

Servings: 2

Ingredients:
- 4 slices deli turkey breast
- 1 avocado, thinly sliced
- 1/4 cup baby spinach leaves

- 1 tablespoon hummus
- Salt and pepper to taste

Directions:
1. Lay out the turkey slices on a clean surface.
2. Spread a thin layer of hummus onto each turkey slice.
3. Place a few baby spinach leaves and avocado slices on top of each turkey slice.
4. Season with salt and pepper to taste.
5. Roll up each turkey slice tightly.
6. Secure with toothpicks if needed.
7. Serve immediately and enjoy these protein-packed turkey and avocado roll-ups!

Nutrition Facts (per serving):
- Calories: 180
- Protein: 15g
- Fat: 10g
- Carbohydrates: 6g
- Fiber: 4g

DESSERTS RECIPES

Banana Almond Chia Pudding

Prep Time: 5 mins

Total Time: 2 hrs 5 mins

Servings: 2

Ingredients:

- 1 ripe banana
- 1 cup almond milk
- 1/4 cup chia seeds
- 1 tablespoon honey or maple syrup
- 1/4 teaspoon vanilla extract
- Optional toppings: sliced almonds, fresh berries

Directions:

1. In a blender, combine the ripe banana, almond milk, honey or maple syrup, and vanilla extract. Blend until smooth.
2. Transfer the banana mixture to a bowl or jar.
3. Stir in the chia seeds until well combined.
4. Cover and refrigerate for at least 2 hours, or until the chia pudding has thickened.
5. Once thickened, stir the chia pudding to evenly distribute the seeds.
6. Serve the chia pudding topped with sliced almonds and fresh berries, if desired.
7. Enjoy this creamy and nutritious banana almond chia pudding as a satisfying dessert or snack!

Nutrition Facts (per serving):
- Calories: 200
- Protein: 5g
- Fat: 8g
- Carbohydrates: 30g
- Fiber: 10g

Avocado Chocolate Mousse

Prep Time: 10 mins

Total Time: 10 mins

Servings: 2

Ingredients:
- 1 ripe avocado
- 2 tablespoons cocoa powder
- 2 tablespoons honey or maple syrup
- 1/4 teaspoon vanilla extract
- Pinch of salt
- Optional toppings: sliced strawberries, shaved dark chocolate

Directions:
1. Scoop the flesh of the ripe avocado into a blender or food processor.
2. Add the cocoa powder, honey or maple syrup, vanilla extract, and a pinch of salt.
3. Blend until smooth and creamy, scraping down the sides as needed.
4. Divide the avocado chocolate mousse into serving glasses.

5. Refrigerate for at least 30 minutes before serving to allow the mousse to set.
6. Serve topped with sliced strawberries and shaved dark chocolate, if desired.
7. Enjoy this rich and indulgent avocado chocolate mousse as a guilt-free dessert option!

Nutrition Facts (per serving):
- Calories: 180
- Protein: 3g
- Fat: 12g
- Carbohydrates: 20g
- Fiber: 7g

Coconut Mango Rice Pudding

Prep Time: 5 mins

Total Time: 25 mins

Servings: 2

Ingredients:
- 1/2 cup cooked rice (such as basmati or jasmine)
- 1 cup coconut milk
- 1 ripe mango, diced
- 2 tablespoons honey or maple syrup
- 1/4 teaspoon vanilla extract
- Pinch of cinnamon
- Optional toppings: toasted coconut flakes, chopped nuts

Directions:
1. In a saucepan, combine the cooked rice and coconut milk.

2. Bring to a simmer over medium heat, stirring occasionally.
3. Once simmering, reduce the heat to low and continue to cook for 15-20 minutes, or until the rice has absorbed the coconut milk and the mixture has thickened.
4. Remove from heat and stir in the diced mango, honey or maple syrup, vanilla extract, and a pinch of cinnamon.
5. Divide the coconut mango rice pudding into serving bowls.
6. Serve warm or chilled, topped with toasted coconut flakes and chopped nuts, if desired.
7. Enjoy this tropical and comforting coconut mango rice pudding as a delightful dessert or snack!

Nutrition Facts (per serving):
- Calories: 250
- Protein: 3g
- Fat: 10g
- Carbohydrates: 40g
- Fiber: 4g

Baked Apples with Cinnamon and Walnuts

Prep Time: 10 mins

Total Time: 40 mins

Servings: 2

Ingredients:
- 2 apples (such as Granny Smith or Honey crisp)
- 2 tablespoons chopped walnuts
- 1 tablespoon honey or maple syrup
- 1/2 teaspoon cinnamon

- Pinch of nutmeg
- 1/4 cup water

Directions:
1. Preheat the oven to 375°F (190°C). Grease a baking dish with non-stick cooking spray.
2. Core the apples and cut a thin slice off the bottom of each apple so they can stand upright.
3. In a small bowl, mix together the chopped walnuts, honey or maple syrup, cinnamon, and nutmeg.
4. Stuff each apple with the walnut mixture, pressing down gently.
5. Place the stuffed apples in the prepared baking dish.
6. Pour the water into the bottom of the baking dish.
7. Bake for 25-30 minutes, or until the apples are tender and lightly browned.
8. Remove from the oven and let cool slightly before serving.
9. Enjoy these warm and comforting baked apples as a wholesome and satisfying dessert!

Nutrition Facts (per serving):
- Calories: 200
- Protein: 2g
- Fat: 5g
- Carbohydrates: 40g
- Fiber: 6g

Frozen Berry Yogurt Bark

Prep Time: 10 mins

Total Time: 3 hrs 10 mins

Servings: 4

Ingredients:

- 1 cup plain Greek yogurt
- 1 tablespoon honey or maple syrup
- 1/2 teaspoon vanilla extract
- 1 cup mixed berries (such as strawberries, blueberries, raspberries)
- 2 tablespoons chopped nuts (such as almonds, walnuts)

Directions:

1. In a mixing bowl, combine the plain Greek yogurt, honey or maple syrup, and vanilla extract. Stir until well combined.
2. Line a baking sheet with parchment paper.
3. Spread the yogurt mixture evenly onto the parchment paper, creating a thin layer.
4. Sprinkle the mixed berries and chopped nuts evenly over the yogurt layer, pressing them gently into the yogurt.
5. Place the baking sheet in the freezer and freeze for at least 3 hours, or until the yogurt bark is completely frozen.
6. Once frozen, remove the baking sheet from the freezer and break the yogurt bark into pieces.
7. Serve immediately and enjoy this refreshing and nutritious frozen berry yogurt bark as a guilt-free dessert or snack!

Nutrition Facts (per serving):

- Calories: 120

- Protein: 6g
- Fat: 5g
- Carbohydrates: 15g
- Fiber: 3g

Chia Seed Pudding with Berries

Prep Time: 5 mins

Total Time: 2 hrs 5 mins

Servings: 2

Ingredients:

- 1/4 cup chia seeds
- 1 cup coconut milk
- 1 tablespoon honey or maple syrup
- 1/2 teaspoon vanilla extract
- 1/2 cup mixed berries (such as strawberries, blueberries, raspberries)
- 2 tablespoons sliced almonds

Directions:

1. In a mixing bowl, combine the chia seeds, coconut milk, honey or maple syrup, and vanilla extract. Stir until well combined.
2. Cover and refrigerate for at least 2 hours, or overnight, to allow the chia pudding to thicken.
3. Once thickened, stir the chia pudding to evenly distribute the seeds.
4. Divide the chia pudding into serving bowls.
5. Top with mixed berries and sliced almonds.

6. Serve chilled and enjoy this creamy and nutritious chia seed pudding as a delightful dessert or snack!

Nutrition Facts (per serving):
- Calories: 220
- Protein: 5g
- Fat: 15g
- Carbohydrates: 20g
- Fiber: 8g

Baked Apple Chips

Prep Time: 10 mins

Total Time: 2 hrs 20 mins

Servings: 2

Ingredients:
- 2 apples (such as Granny Smith or Honey crisp)
- 1 tablespoon honey or maple syrup
- 1/2 teaspoon ground cinnamon

Directions:
1. Preheat the oven to 200°F (95°C). Line a baking sheet with parchment paper.
2. Core the apples and thinly slice them using a mandolin or sharp knife.
3. In a small bowl, whisk together the honey or maple syrup and ground cinnamon.
4. Arrange the apple slices in a single layer on the prepared baking sheet.
5. Brush the apple slices with the honey or maple syrup mixture.

6. Bake for 2 hours, flipping the apple slices halfway through, or until they are crispy and golden brown.
7. Remove from the oven and let cool completely before serving.
8. Enjoy these crunchy and naturally sweet baked apple chips as a healthy dessert or snack option!

Nutrition Facts (per serving):
- Calories: 120
- Protein: 1g
- Fat: 0g
- Carbohydrates: 30g
- Fiber: 5g

Coconut Banana Ice Cream

Prep Time: 5 mins

Total Time: 4 hrs 5 mins

Servings: 2

Ingredients:
- 2 ripe bananas, sliced and frozen
- 1/4 cup coconut milk
- 2 tablespoons shredded coconut
- 1 tablespoon honey or maple syrup (optional)

Directions:
1. Place the frozen banana slices, coconut milk, shredded coconut, and honey or maple syrup (if using) in a blender or food processor.
2. Blend until smooth and creamy, scraping down the sides as needed.

3. Transfer the mixture to a freezer-safe container and freeze for at least 4 hours, or until firm.
4. Once frozen, scoop the coconut banana ice cream into serving bowls.
5. Serve immediately and enjoy this creamy and naturally sweet ice cream as a refreshing dessert!

Nutrition Facts (per serving):
- Calories: 150
- Protein: 2g
- Fat: 5g
- Carbohydrates: 30g
- Fiber: 4g

Chocolate Avocado Mousse

Prep Time: 10 mins

Total Time: 10 mins

Servings: 2

Ingredients:
- 1 ripe avocado
- 2 tablespoons cocoa powder
- 2 tablespoons honey or maple syrup
- 1/2 teaspoon vanilla extract
- Pinch of salt

Directions:
1. Scoop the flesh of the ripe avocado into a blender or food processor.

2. Add the cocoa powder, honey or maple syrup, vanilla extract, and a pinch of salt.
3. Blend until smooth and creamy, scraping down the sides as needed.
4. Divide the chocolate avocado mousse into serving glasses.
5. Serve immediately and enjoy this rich and indulgent chocolate mousse as a guilt-free dessert option!

Nutrition Facts (per serving):
- Calories: 200
- Protein: 3g
- Fat: 12g
- Carbohydrates: 20g
- Fiber: 7g

Cinnamon Baked Pears

Prep Time: 10 mins
Total Time: 30 mins
Servings: 2

Ingredients:
- 2 ripe pears, halved and cored
- 1 tablespoon honey or maple syrup
- 1/2 teaspoon ground cinnamon
- 2 tablespoons chopped walnuts or pecans

Directions:
1. Preheat the oven to 375°F (190°C). Grease a baking dish with non-stick cooking spray.
2. Place the pear halves, cut side up, in the prepared baking dish.

3. Drizzle the honey or maple syrup over the pear halves.
4. Sprinkle ground cinnamon evenly over the pear halves.
5. Top each pear half with chopped walnuts or pecans.
6. Bake for 20-25 minutes, or until the pears are tender and golden brown.
7. Remove from the oven and let cool slightly before serving.
8. Enjoy these warm and fragrant cinnamon baked pears as a comforting and wholesome dessert!

Nutrition Facts (per serving):
- Calories: 160
- Protein: 2g
- Fat: 5g
- Carbohydrates: 30g
- Fiber: 6g

Coconut Chia Pudding with Fresh Fruit

Prep Time: 5 mins

Total Time: 2 hrs 5 mins

Servings: 2

Ingredients:
- 1/4 cup chia seeds
- 1 cup coconut milk
- 1 tablespoon honey or maple syrup
- 1/2 teaspoon vanilla extract
- 1/2 cup mixed fresh fruit (such as berries, mango, kiwi)
- 2 tablespoons unsweetened shredded coconut

Directions:

1. In a mixing bowl, combine the chia seeds, coconut milk, honey or maple syrup, and vanilla extract. Stir until well combined.
2. Cover and refrigerate for at least 2 hours, or overnight, to allow the chia pudding to thicken.
3. Once thickened, stir the chia pudding to evenly distribute the seeds.
4. Divide the chia pudding into serving bowls.
5. Top with mixed fresh fruit and shredded coconut.
6. Serve chilled and enjoy this creamy and nutritious coconut chia pudding as a delightful dessert or snack!

Nutrition Facts (per serving):
- Calories: 220
- Protein: 5g
- Fat: 15g
- Carbohydrates: 20g
- Fiber: 8g

Almond Flour Banana Bread

Prep Time: 15 mins

Total Time: 1 hr 15 mins

Servings: 8

Ingredients:
- 2 ripe bananas, mashed
- 2 eggs
- 1/4 cup honey or maple syrup
- 1/4 cup coconut oil, melted
- 1 teaspoon vanilla extract

- 2 cups almond flour
- 1 teaspoon baking powder
- 1/2 teaspoon ground cinnamon
- Pinch of salt
- Optional add-ins: chopped nuts, dried fruit

Directions:

1. Preheat the oven to 350°F (175°C). Grease a loaf pan with coconut oil or line with parchment paper.
2. In a large mixing bowl, combine the mashed bananas, eggs, honey or maple syrup, melted coconut oil, and vanilla extract. Mix until well combined.
3. Add the almond flour, baking powder, ground cinnamon, and salt to the wet ingredients. Stir until just combined.
4. If desired, fold in chopped nuts or dried fruit.
5. Pour the batter into the prepared loaf pan and spread it out evenly.
6. Bake for 50-60 minutes, or until a toothpick inserted into the center comes out clean.
7. Remove from the oven and let cool in the pan for 10 minutes before transferring to a wire rack to cool completely.
8. Slice and enjoy this delicious almond flour banana bread as a satisfying and wholesome dessert or snack!

Nutrition Facts (per serving):

- Calories: 250
- Protein: 7g
- Fat: 18g

- Carbohydrates: 20g
- Fiber: 4g

Baked Coconut Mango Oatmeal Cups

Prep Time: 10 mins

Total Time: 30 mins

Servings: 6

Ingredients:

- 1 cup rolled oats
- 1/4 cup unsweetened shredded coconut
- 1 ripe banana, mashed
- 1/2 cup coconut milk
- 1/4 cup honey or maple syrup
- 1/2 teaspoon vanilla extract
- 1/2 cup diced mango
- 2 tablespoons chopped nuts (such as almonds or walnuts)

Directions:

1. Preheat the oven to 350°F (175°C). Grease a muffin tin with coconut oil or line with silicone baking cups.
2. In a mixing bowl, combine the rolled oats, shredded coconut, mashed banana, coconut milk, honey or maple syrup, and vanilla extract. Mix until well combined.
3. Fold in the diced mango and chopped nuts.
4. Divide the oatmeal mixture evenly among the muffin cups.
5. Bake for 20-25 minutes, or until the oatmeal cups are set and lightly golden brown.

6. Remove from the oven and let cool in the muffin tin for 5 minutes before transferring to a wire rack to cool completely.
7. Serve these baked coconut mango oatmeal cups warm or at room temperature as a delicious and nutritious dessert or snack!

Nutrition Facts (per serving):
- Calories: 180
- Protein: 4g
- Fat: 7g
- Carbohydrates: 26g
- Fiber: 3g

Chocolate Peanut Butter Protein Balls

Prep Time: 15 mins

Total Time: 1 hr. 15 mins

Servings: 12

Ingredients:
- 1 cup rolled oats
- 1/2 cup natural peanut butter
- 1/4 cup honey or maple syrup
- 2 tablespoons cocoa powder
- 1/4 cup chocolate protein powder
- 1/4 cup unsweetened shredded coconut (optional)
- 2 tablespoons mini chocolate chips (optional)

Directions:
1. In a mixing bowl, combine the rolled oats, peanut butter, honey or maple syrup, cocoa powder, chocolate protein powder,

shredded coconut (if using), and mini chocolate chips (if using). Mix until well combined.
2. If the mixture is too dry, add a little more peanut butter or honey/maple syrup. If it's too wet, add more rolled oats.
3. Roll the mixture into bite-sized balls using your hands.
4. Place the protein balls on a baking sheet lined with parchment paper.
5. Refrigerate for at least 1 hour, or until firm.
6. Once firm, transfer the protein balls to an airtight container and store in the refrigerator until ready to eat.
7. Enjoy these chocolate peanut butter protein balls as a delicious and protein-rich dessert or snack!

Nutrition Facts (per serving - 1 ball):
- Calories: 130
- Protein: 5g
- Fat: 7g
- Carbohydrates: 13g
- Fiber: 2g

Apple Cinnamon Quinoa Breakfast Bars

Prep Time: 15 mins

Total Time: 40 mins

Servings: 9 bars

Ingredients:
- 1 cup cooked quinoa
- 1 large apple, peeled and grated
- 1/4 cup almond butter

- 1/4 cup honey or maple syrup
- 1 teaspoon ground cinnamon
- 1/4 teaspoon ground nutmeg
- 1/4 teaspoon salt
- 1/4 cup chopped nuts (such as walnuts or pecans)
- 1/4 cup dried cranberries or raisins

Directions:

1. Preheat the oven to 350°F (175°C). Grease a square baking dish or line it with parchment paper.
2. In a large mixing bowl, combine the cooked quinoa, grated apple, almond butter, honey or maple syrup, ground cinnamon, ground nutmeg, and salt. Mix until well combined.
3. Fold in the chopped nuts and dried cranberries or raisins.
4. Transfer the mixture to the prepared baking dish and press it down evenly with a spatula.
5. Bake for 25-30 minutes, or until the edges are golden brown and the bars are set.
6. Remove from the oven and let cool completely in the baking dish before slicing into bars.
7. Enjoy these apple cinnamon quinoa breakfast bars as a nutritious and satisfying dessert or snack option!

Nutrition Facts (per serving):

- Calories: 160
- Protein: 4g
- Fat: 7g
- Carbohydrates: 22g

- Fiber: 3g

Berry Avocado Parfait

Prep Time: 10 mins

Total Time: 10 mins

Servings: 2

Ingredients:

- 1 ripe avocado
- 1 cup mixed berries (such as strawberries, blueberries, raspberries)
- 1/4 cup unsweetened Greek yogurt or dairy-free yogurt alternative
- 2 tablespoons honey or maple syrup
- 1/4 cup granola
- Fresh mint leaves for garnish (optional)

Directions:

1. Scoop the flesh of the ripe avocado into a blender or food processor.
2. Add the mixed berries, Greek yogurt or dairy-free yogurt alternative, and honey or maple syrup to the blender.
3. Blend until smooth and creamy, scraping down the sides as needed.
4. Divide the berry avocado mixture into serving glasses.
5. Top each glass with a layer of granola.
6. Garnish with fresh mint leaves, if desired.
7. Serve immediately and enjoy this refreshing and nutritious berry avocado parfait as a delightful dessert or snack!

Nutrition Facts (per serving):
- Calories: 250
- Protein: 6g
- Fat: 12g
- Carbohydrates: 32g
- Fiber: 7g

Pumpkin Spice Chia Seed Pudding

Prep Time: 5 mins

Total Time: 2 hrs 5 mins

Servings: 2

Ingredients:
- 1/4 cup chia seeds
- 1 cup unsweetened almond milk or coconut milk
- 1/4 cup pumpkin puree
- 2 tablespoons honey or maple syrup
- 1/2 teaspoon vanilla extract
- 1/2 teaspoon ground cinnamon
- 1/4 teaspoon ground ginger
- Pinch of ground nutmeg
- Pinch of ground cloves
- 2 tablespoons chopped pecans or walnuts (optional)
- Whipped coconut cream for topping (optional)

Directions:
1. In a mixing bowl, combine the chia seeds, almond milk or coconut milk, pumpkin puree, honey or maple syrup, vanilla

extract, ground cinnamon, ground ginger, ground nutmeg, and ground cloves. Stir until well combined.
2. Cover and refrigerate for at least 2 hours, or overnight, to allow the chia pudding to thicken.
3. Once thickened, stir the chia pudding to evenly distribute the seeds.
4. Divide the pumpkin spice chia seed pudding into serving bowls.
5. Top with chopped pecans or walnuts and whipped coconut cream, if desired.
6. Serve chilled and enjoy this creamy and flavorful pumpkin spice chia seed pudding as a delicious dessert or snack!

Nutrition Facts (per serving):
- Calories: 220
- Protein: 6g
- Fat: 12g
- Carbohydrates: 25g
- Fiber: 9g

Coconut Mango Rice Pudding

Prep Time: 10 mins
Total Time: 40 mins
Servings: 4

Ingredients:
- 1/2 cup Arborio rice
- 1 can (13.5 oz) coconut milk
- 1 cup water
- 2 tablespoons honey or maple syrup

- 1/2 teaspoon vanilla extract
- 1 ripe mango, diced
- Unsweetened shredded coconut for garnish (optional)

Directions:
1. In a saucepan, combine the Arborio rice, coconut milk, water, honey or maple syrup, and vanilla extract. Stir well.
2. Bring the mixture to a boil over medium heat.
3. Reduce the heat to low, cover, and simmer for 25-30 minutes, stirring occasionally, until the rice is tender and the mixture has thickened.
4. Remove from heat and let cool slightly.
5. Divide the coconut mango rice pudding into serving bowls.
6. Top with diced mango and shredded coconut, if desired.
7. Serve warm or chilled and enjoy this creamy and tropical coconut mango rice pudding as a delightful dessert!

Nutrition Facts (per serving):
- Calories: 290
- Protein: 4g
- Fat: 18g
- Carbohydrates: 31g
- Fiber: 2g

Dark Chocolate Avocado Mousse

Prep Time: 10 mins

Total Time: 10 mins

Servings: 2

Ingredients:

- 1 ripe avocado
- 2 tablespoons cocoa powder
- 2 tablespoons honey or maple syrup
- 1/2 teaspoon vanilla extract
- Pinch of salt
- Dark chocolate shavings for garnish (optional)

Directions:
1. Scoop the flesh of the ripe avocado into a blender or food processor.
2. Add the cocoa powder, honey or maple syrup, vanilla extract, and a pinch of salt to the blender.
3. Blend until smooth and creamy, scraping down the sides as needed.
4. Divide the dark chocolate avocado mousse into serving glasses.
5. Garnish with dark chocolate shavings, if desired.
6. Serve immediately and enjoy this rich and decadent dark chocolate avocado mousse as a guilt-free dessert or snack!

Nutrition Facts (per serving):
- Calories: 200
- Protein: 3g
- Fat: 14g
- Carbohydrates: 20g
- Fiber: 7g

Banana Oatmeal Cookies

Prep Time: 10 mins

Total Time: 20 mins

Servings: 12 cookies

Ingredients:

- 2 ripe bananas, mashed
- 1 cup rolled oats
- 1/4 cup almond flour
- 2 tablespoons honey or maple syrup
- 1/4 teaspoon ground cinnamon
- 1/4 teaspoon vanilla extract
- Pinch of salt
- 2 tablespoons dark chocolate chips (optional)
- 2 tablespoons chopped nuts (such as walnuts or almonds) (optional)

Directions:

1. Preheat the oven to 350°F (175°C). Line a baking sheet with parchment paper.
2. In a mixing bowl, combine the mashed bananas, rolled oats, almond flour, honey or maple syrup, ground cinnamon, vanilla extract, and a pinch of salt. Mix until well combined.
3. If desired, fold in dark chocolate chips and chopped nuts.
4. Drop spoonfuls of the cookie dough onto the prepared baking sheet, spacing them apart.
5. Flatten each cookie slightly with the back of a spoon.
6. Bake for 10-12 minutes, or until the cookies are golden brown around the edges.

7. Remove from the oven and let cool on the baking sheet for 5 minutes before transferring to a wire rack to cool completely.
8. Enjoy these banana oatmeal cookies as a wholesome and satisfying dessert or snack option!

Nutrition Facts (per serving - 1 cookie):
- Calories: 80
- Protein: 2g
- Fat: 2g
- Carbohydrates: 15g
- Fiber: 2g

SOUP RECIPES

Creamy Butternut Squash Soup

Prep Time: 15 mins

Total Time: 40 mins

Servings: 4

Ingredients:

- 1 medium butternut squash, peeled, seeded, and cubed
- 1 onion, chopped
- 2 cloves garlic, minced
- 4 cups vegetable broth
- 1/2 teaspoon ground cinnamon
- 1/4 teaspoon ground nutmeg
- Salt and pepper to taste
- 1/2 cup coconut milk or almond milk
- Fresh parsley or chives for garnish (optional)

Directions:

1. In a large pot, heat some olive oil over medium heat. Add the chopped onion and minced garlic, and sauté until softened, about 5 minutes.
2. Add the cubed butternut squash to the pot, along with the vegetable broth, ground cinnamon, ground nutmeg, salt, and pepper. Bring to a boil.
3. Reduce the heat to low, cover, and simmer for 20-25 minutes, or until the squash is tender.

4. Use an immersion blender to blend the soup until smooth. Alternatively, transfer the soup to a blender and blend in batches until smooth.
5. Stir in the coconut milk or almond milk until well combined.
6. Taste and adjust seasoning if needed.
7. Ladle the soup into bowls and garnish with fresh parsley or chives, if desired.
8. Serve hot and enjoy this creamy and comforting butternut squash soup!

Nutrition Facts (per serving):
- Calories: 120
- Protein: 2g
- Fat: 3g
- Carbohydrates: 24g
- Fiber: 5g

Lentil and Vegetable Soup

Prep Time: 15 mins

Total Time: 45 mins

Servings: 6

Ingredients:
- 1 cup dried green lentils, rinsed and drained
- 1 onion, chopped
- 2 carrots, diced
- 2 celery stalks, diced
- 2 cloves garlic, minced
- 4 cups vegetable broth

- 1 can (14 oz) diced tomatoes
- 1 teaspoon ground cumin
- 1 teaspoon ground coriander
- 1/2 teaspoon smoked paprika
- Salt and pepper to taste
- Fresh parsley or cilantro for garnish (optional)

Directions:

1. In a large pot, heat some olive oil over medium heat. Add the chopped onion, diced carrots, diced celery, and minced garlic, and sauté until softened, about 5 minutes.
2. Add the rinsed lentils, vegetable broth, diced tomatoes (with their juices), ground cumin, ground coriander, smoked paprika, salt, and pepper to the pot. Stir to combine.
3. Bring the soup to a boil, then reduce the heat to low, cover, and simmer for 25-30 minutes, or until the lentils are tender.
4. Taste and adjust seasoning if needed.
5. Ladle the soup into bowls and garnish with fresh parsley or cilantro, if desired.
6. Serve hot and enjoy this hearty and nutritious lentil and vegetable soup!

Nutrition Facts (per serving):

- Calories: 180
- Protein: 10g
- Fat: 1g
- Carbohydrates: 32g
- Fiber: 12g

Roasted Tomato Basil Soup

Prep Time: 10 mins

Total Time: 50 mins

Servings: 4

Ingredients:

- 2 lbs ripe tomatoes, halved
- 1 onion, chopped
- 3 cloves garlic, minced
- 2 tablespoons olive oil
- 4 cups vegetable broth
- 1/4 cup fresh basil leaves, chopped
- Salt and pepper to taste
- Balsamic glaze for garnish (optional)

Directions:

1. Preheat the oven to 400°F (200°C). Place the halved tomatoes on a baking sheet, cut side up. Drizzle with olive oil and season with salt and pepper.
2. Roast the tomatoes in the preheated oven for 30-35 minutes, or until softened and slightly caramelized.
3. In a large pot, heat some olive oil over medium heat. Add the chopped onion and minced garlic, and sauté until softened, about 5 minutes.
4. Add the roasted tomatoes (including any juices) to the pot, along with the vegetable broth and chopped basil. Bring to a boil.

5. Reduce the heat to low, cover, and simmer for 10-15 minutes to allow the flavors to meld together.
6. Use an immersion blender to blend the soup until smooth. Alternatively, transfer the soup to a blender and blend in batches until smooth.
7. Taste and adjust seasoning if needed.
8. Ladle the soup into bowls and drizzle with balsamic glaze, if desired.
9. Serve hot and enjoy this rich and flavorful roasted tomato basil soup!

Nutrition Facts (per serving):
- Calories: 150
- Protein: 3g
- Fat: 7g
- Carbohydrates: 20g
- Fiber: 5g

Ginger Carrot Soup

Prep Time: 10 mins
Total Time: 35 mins
Servings: 4

Ingredients:
- 1 lb carrots, peeled and chopped
- 1 onion, chopped
- 2 cloves garlic, minced
- 2 tablespoons fresh ginger, grated
- 4 cups vegetable broth

- 1/2 cup coconut milk or almond milk
- 1 tablespoon olive oil
- Salt and pepper to taste
- Fresh cilantro for garnish (optional)

Directions:

1. In a large pot, heat some olive oil over medium heat. Add the chopped onion, minced garlic, and grated ginger, and sauté until fragrant, about 2 minutes.
2. Add the chopped carrots to the pot and sauté for another 5 minutes.
3. Pour in the vegetable broth and bring to a boil. Reduce the heat to low, cover, and simmer for 20-25 minutes, or until the carrots are tender.
4. Use an immersion blender to blend the soup until smooth. Alternatively, transfer the soup to a blender and blend in batches until smooth.
5. Stir in the coconut milk or almond milk until well combined.
6. Taste and adjust seasoning if needed.
7. Ladle the soup into bowls and garnish with fresh cilantro, if desired.
8. Serve hot and enjoy this warming and comforting ginger carrot soup!

Nutrition Facts (per serving):

- Calories: 120
- Protein: 2g
- Fat: 5g

- Carbohydrates: 18g
- Fiber: 5g

Creamy Mushroom Soup

Prep Time: 10 mins

Total Time: 30 mins

Servings: 4

Ingredients:

- 1 lb mushrooms, sliced (button mushrooms or cremini mushrooms)
- 1 onion, chopped
- 2 cloves garlic, minced
- 4 cups vegetable broth
- 1/2 cup coconut milk or almond milk
- 2 tablespoons olive oil
- 2 tablespoons all-purpose flour or gluten-free flour
- Salt and pepper to taste
- Fresh thyme for garnish (optional)

Directions:

1. In a large pot, heat some olive oil over medium heat. Add the chopped onion and minced garlic, and sauté until softened, about 5 minutes.
2. Add the sliced mushrooms to the pot and sauté until they release their moisture and start to brown, about 8-10 minutes.
3. Sprinkle the flour over the mushrooms and stir to coat.
4. Pour in the vegetable broth and bring to a boil. Reduce the heat to low, cover, and simmer for 10-15 minutes.

5. Use an immersion blender to blend the soup until smooth. Alternatively, transfer the soup to a blender and blend in batches until smooth.
6. Stir in the coconut milk or almond milk until well combined.
7. Taste and adjust seasoning if needed.
8. Ladle the soup into bowls and garnish with fresh thyme, if desired.
9. Serve hot and enjoy this creamy and flavorful mushroom soup!

Nutrition Facts (per serving):
- Calories: 140
- Protein: 4g
- Fat: 8g
- Carbohydrates: 14g
- Fiber: 3g

These soup recipes offer nourishing and flavorful options suitable for individuals with EPI, providing a comforting and satisfying meal choice.

Spicy Black Bean Soup

Prep Time: 10 mins

Total Time: 30 mins

Servings: 4

Ingredients:
- 2 cans (15 oz each) black beans, drained and rinsed
- 1 onion, chopped
- 2 cloves garlic, minced
- 1 bell pepper, diced

- 1 jalapeño pepper, diced (seeds removed for less heat)
- 4 cups vegetable broth
- 1 teaspoon ground cumin
- 1 teaspoon chili powder
- 1/2 teaspoon smoked paprika
- Salt and pepper to taste
- Juice of 1 lime
- Fresh cilantro for garnish (optional)
- Avocado slices for garnish (optional)
- Tortilla chips or strips for serving (optional)

Directions:

1. In a large pot, heat some olive oil over medium heat. Add the chopped onion, minced garlic, diced bell pepper, and diced jalapeño pepper, and sauté until softened, about 5 minutes.
2. Add the drained and rinsed black beans to the pot, along with the vegetable broth, ground cumin, chili powder, smoked paprika, salt, and pepper. Stir to combine.
3. Bring the soup to a boil, then reduce the heat to low, cover, and simmer for 15-20 minutes to allow the flavors to meld together.
4. Use an immersion blender to blend a portion of the soup until smooth, leaving some chunks of beans and vegetables for texture. Alternatively, transfer a portion of the soup to a blender and blend until smooth, then return it to the pot.
5. Stir in the lime juice until well combined.
6. Taste and adjust seasoning if needed.

7. Ladle the soup into bowls and garnish with fresh cilantro, avocado slices, and tortilla chips or strips, if desired.
8. Serve hot and enjoy this hearty and flavorful spicy black bean soup!

Nutrition Facts (per serving):
- Calories: 220
- Protein: 10g
- Fat: 2g
- Carbohydrates: 40g
- Fiber: 12g

Butternut Squash Soup

Prep Time: 15 mins

Total Time: 45 mins

Servings: 4

Ingredients:
- 1 medium butternut squash, peeled, seeded, and diced
- 1 onion, chopped
- 2 cloves garlic, minced
- 1 carrot, peeled and chopped
- 4 cups vegetable broth
- 1 teaspoon dried thyme
- 1/2 teaspoon ground cinnamon
- Salt and pepper to taste
- 2 tablespoons olive oil
- Fresh parsley for garnish (optional)
- Pumpkin seeds for garnish (optional)

Directions:
1. Heat olive oil in a large pot over medium heat. Add the chopped onion, minced garlic, and chopped carrot. Sauté until softened, about 5 minutes.
2. Add the diced butternut squash to the pot along with the vegetable broth, dried thyme, ground cinnamon, salt, and pepper. Bring to a boil, then reduce heat to low, cover, and simmer for 25-30 minutes until the squash is tender.
3. Use an immersion blender to blend the soup until smooth. Alternatively, transfer the soup to a blender and blend in batches until smooth.
4. Taste and adjust seasoning if needed.
5. Ladle the soup into bowls and garnish with fresh parsley and pumpkin seeds, if desired.
6. Serve hot and enjoy this creamy and comforting butternut squash soup!

Nutrition Facts (per serving):
- Calories: 180
- Protein: 3g
- Fat: 7g
- Carbohydrates: 30g
- Fiber: 6g

Lentil Soup

Prep Time: 10 mins
Total Time: 40 mins
Servings: 4

Ingredients:

- 1 cup dried green or brown lentils, rinsed
- 1 onion, chopped
- 2 cloves garlic, minced
- 1 carrot, peeled and chopped
- 1 stalk celery, chopped
- 4 cups vegetable broth
- 1 can (14 oz) diced tomatoes
- 1 teaspoon ground cumin
- 1 teaspoon paprika
- Salt and pepper to taste
- Fresh parsley for garnish (optional)
- Lemon wedges for serving (optional)

Directions:

1. In a large pot, heat some olive oil over medium heat. Add the chopped onion, minced garlic, chopped carrot, and chopped celery. Sauté until softened, about 5 minutes.
2. Add the rinsed lentils, vegetable broth, diced tomatoes, ground cumin, paprika, salt, and pepper to the pot. Bring to a boil, then reduce heat to low, cover, and simmer for 25-30 minutes until the lentils are tender.
3. Taste and adjust seasoning if needed.
4. Ladle the soup into bowls and garnish with fresh parsley. Serve with lemon wedges on the side for a burst of freshness, if desired.
5. Serve hot and enjoy this hearty and nutritious lentil soup!

Nutrition Facts (per serving):

- Calories: 220
- Protein: 12g
- Fat: 1g
- Carbohydrates: 40g
- Fiber: 15g

Tomato Basil Soup

Prep Time: 10 mins

Total Time: 35 mins

Servings: 4

Ingredients:

- 1 tablespoon olive oil
- 1 onion, chopped
- 2 cloves garlic, minced
- 2 cans (14 oz each) diced tomatoes
- 2 cups vegetable broth
- 1 teaspoon dried basil
- 1/2 teaspoon dried oregano
- Salt and pepper to taste
- 1/4 cup coconut milk or almond milk (optional, for creaminess)
- Fresh basil leaves for garnish (optional)
- Croutons for serving (optional)

Directions:

1. Heat olive oil in a large pot over medium heat. Add the chopped onion and minced garlic, and sauté until softened, about 5 minutes.

2. Add the diced tomatoes (with their juices), vegetable broth, dried basil, dried oregano, salt, and pepper to the pot. Bring to a boil, then reduce heat to low, cover, and simmer for 20-25 minutes.
3. Use an immersion blender to blend the soup until smooth. Alternatively, transfer the soup to a blender and blend in batches until smooth.
4. Stir in the coconut milk or almond milk if using, until well combined.
5. Taste and adjust seasoning if needed.
6. Ladle the soup into bowls and garnish with fresh basil leaves and croutons, if desired.
7. Serve hot and enjoy this classic and comforting tomato basil soup!

Nutrition Facts (per serving):
- Calories: 120
- Protein: 3g
- Fat: 3g
- Carbohydrates: 20g
- Fiber: 5g

Carrot Ginger Soup

Prep Time: 10 mins

Total Time: 35 mins

Servings: 4

Ingredients:
- 1 tablespoon olive oil

- 1 onion, chopped
- 2 cloves garlic, minced
- 1 tablespoon fresh ginger, minced
- 4 cups chopped carrots
- 4 cups vegetable broth
- 1/2 teaspoon ground turmeric
- Salt and pepper to taste
- Coconut cream or yogurt for serving (optional)
- Fresh cilantro for garnish (optional)

Directions:

1. In a large pot, heat olive oil over medium heat. Add the chopped onion, minced garlic, and minced ginger, and sauté until fragrant, about 2 minutes.
2. Add the chopped carrots to the pot and sauté for another 5 minutes.
3. Pour in the vegetable broth, ground turmeric, salt, and pepper. Bring to a boil, then reduce heat to low, cover, and simmer for 20-25 minutes until the carrots are tender.
4. Use an immersion blender to blend the soup until smooth. Alternatively, transfer the soup to a blender and blend in batches until smooth.
5. Taste and adjust seasoning if needed.
6. Ladle the soup into bowls and drizzle with coconut cream or yogurt, if using. Garnish with fresh cilantro, if desired.
7. Serve hot and enjoy this vibrant and flavorful carrot ginger soup!

Nutrition Facts (per serving):

- Calories: 110
- Protein: 2g
- Fat: 4g
- Carbohydrates: 18g
- Fiber: 5g

Spinach and Potato Soup

Prep Time: 15 mins

Total Time: 40 mins

Servings: 4

Ingredients:

- 1 tablespoon olive oil
- 1 onion, chopped
- 2 cloves garlic, minced
- 2 large potatoes, peeled and diced
- 4 cups vegetable broth
- 4 cups fresh spinach leaves
- 1/2 teaspoon dried thyme
- Salt and pepper to taste
- Lemon wedges for serving (optional)

Directions:

1. Heat olive oil in a large pot over medium heat. Add the chopped onion and minced garlic, and sauté until softened, about 5 minutes.
2. Add the diced potatoes to the pot and sauté for another 5 minutes.

3. Pour in the vegetable broth and bring to a boil. Reduce heat to low, cover, and simmer for 15-20 minutes until the potatoes are tender.
4. Stir in the fresh spinach leaves and dried thyme. Cook for an additional 5 minutes until the spinach is wilted.
5. Use an immersion blender to blend a portion of the soup until smooth, leaving some chunks of potatoes and spinach for texture. Alternatively, transfer a portion of the soup to a blender and blend until smooth, then return it to the pot.
6. Taste and adjust seasoning if needed.
7. Ladle the soup into bowls and serve with lemon wedges on the side for a fresh squeeze of flavor, if desired.
8. Serve hot and enjoy this nutritious and comforting spinach and potato soup!

Nutrition Facts (per serving):
- Calories: 160
- Protein: 4g
- Fat: 3g
- Carbohydrates: 30g
- Fiber: 5g

Vegetable Quinoa Soup

Prep Time: 10 mins

Total Time: 35 mins

Servings: 4

Ingredients:
- 1 tablespoon olive oil

- 1 onion, diced
- 2 cloves garlic, minced
- 2 carrots, peeled and diced
- 2 celery stalks, diced
- 1 bell pepper, diced
- 1 cup quinoa, rinsed
- 6 cups vegetable broth
- 1 teaspoon dried thyme
- Salt and pepper to taste
- Fresh parsley for garnish (optional)

Directions:

1. In a large pot, heat olive oil over medium heat. Add the diced onion and minced garlic, and sauté until softened, about 5 minutes.
2. Add the diced carrots, celery, and bell pepper to the pot. Cook for another 5 minutes until the vegetables are slightly softened.
3. Stir in the rinsed quinoa, vegetable broth, dried thyme, salt, and pepper. Bring to a boil, then reduce heat to low, cover, and simmer for 20 minutes until the quinoa is cooked and the vegetables are tender.
4. Taste and adjust seasoning if needed.
5. Ladle the soup into bowls and garnish with fresh parsley, if desired.
6. Serve hot and enjoy this hearty and nutritious vegetable quinoa soup!

Nutritional Information (per serving):

- Calories: 250
- Protein: 8g
- Fat: 5g
- Carbohydrates: 45g
- Fiber: 8g

Creamy Cauliflower Soup

Prep Time: 10 mins
Total Time: 35 mins
Servings: 4

Ingredients:
- 1 tablespoon olive oil
- 1 onion, chopped
- 2 cloves garlic, minced
- 1 head cauliflower, chopped into florets
- 4 cups vegetable broth
- 1/2 teaspoon dried thyme
- Salt and pepper to taste
- 1/2 cup coconut milk (from a can)
- Fresh chives for garnish (optional)

Directions:
1. Heat olive oil in a large pot over medium heat. Add the chopped onion and minced garlic, and sauté until softened, about 5 minutes.
2. Add the cauliflower florets to the pot along with the vegetable broth, dried thyme, salt, and pepper. Bring to a boil, then reduce

heat to low, cover, and simmer for 20 minutes until the cauliflower is tender.
3. Use an immersion blender to blend the soup until smooth. Alternatively, transfer the soup to a blender and blend in batches until smooth.
4. Stir in the coconut milk until well combined and heated through.
5. Taste and adjust seasoning if needed.
6. Ladle the soup into bowls and garnish with fresh chives, if desired.
7. Serve hot and enjoy this creamy and delicious cauliflower soup!

Nutritional Information (per serving):
- Calories: 180
- Protein: 5g
- Fat: 10g
- Carbohydrates: 20g
- Fiber: 5g

Lentil and Vegetable Soup

Prep Time: 10 mins

Total Time: 45 mins

Servings: 4

Ingredients:
- 1 tablespoon olive oil
- 1 onion, diced
- 2 cloves garlic, minced
- 1 carrot, diced

- 1 celery stalk, diced
- 1 cup dried lentils, rinsed
- 4 cups vegetable broth
- 1 teaspoon ground cumin
- 1/2 teaspoon paprika
- Salt and pepper to taste
- Fresh parsley for garnish (optional)

Directions:

1. Heat olive oil in a large pot over medium heat. Add the diced onion and minced garlic, and sauté until softened, about 5 minutes.
2. Add the diced carrot and celery to the pot, and cook for another 5 minutes until slightly softened.
3. Stir in the rinsed lentils, vegetable broth, ground cumin, paprika, salt, and pepper. Bring to a boil, then reduce heat to low, cover, and simmer for 30 minutes until the lentils are tender.
4. Taste and adjust seasoning if needed.
5. Ladle the soup into bowls and garnish with fresh parsley, if desired.
6. Serve hot and enjoy this hearty and nutritious lentil and vegetable soup!

Nutritional Information (per serving):

- Calories: 220
- Protein: 12g
- Fat: 3g

- Carbohydrates: 35g
- Fiber: 12g

Butternut Squash Soup

Prep Time: 15 mins

Total Time: 40 mins

Servings: 4

Ingredients:

- 1 tablespoon olive oil
- 1 onion, chopped
- 2 cloves garlic, minced
- 1 medium butternut squash, peeled, seeded, and chopped
- 4 cups vegetable broth
- 1 teaspoon ground cinnamon
- 1/2 teaspoon ground nutmeg
- Salt and pepper to taste
- Coconut cream for serving (optional)
- Fresh thyme for garnish (optional)

Directions:

1. In a large pot, heat olive oil over medium heat. Add the chopped onion and minced garlic, and sauté until softened, about 5 minutes.
2. Add the chopped butternut squash to the pot along with the vegetable broth, ground cinnamon, ground nutmeg, salt, and pepper. Bring to a boil, then reduce heat to low, cover, and simmer for 20 minutes until the squash is tender.

3. Use an immersion blender to blend the soup until smooth. Alternatively, transfer the soup to a blender and blend in batches until smooth.
4. Taste and adjust seasoning if needed.
5. Ladle the soup into bowls and swirl in some coconut cream, if using. Garnish with fresh thyme, if desired.
6. Serve hot and enjoy this velvety and comforting butternut squash soup!

Nutritional Information (per serving):
- Calories: 180
- Protein: 3g
- Fat: 5g
- Carbohydrates: 35g
- Fiber: 6g

Tomato Basil Soup

Prep Time: 10 mins

Total Time: 30 mins

Servings: 4

Ingredients:
- 1 tablespoon olive oil
- 1 onion, chopped
- 2 cloves garlic, minced
- 2 cans (14 oz each) diced tomatoes
- 2 cups vegetable broth
- 1 teaspoon dried basil
- 1/2 teaspoon dried oregano

- Salt and pepper to taste
- Fresh basil leaves for garnish (optional)
- Croutons for serving (optional)

Directions:

1. Heat olive oil in a large pot over medium heat. Add the chopped onion and minced garlic, and sauté until softened, about 5 minutes.
2. Add the diced tomatoes (with their juices) to the pot along with the vegetable broth, dried basil, dried oregano, salt, and pepper. Bring to a boil, then reduce heat to low, cover, and simmer for 15 minutes.
3. Use an immersion blender to blend the soup until smooth. Alternatively, transfer the soup to a blender and blend in batches until smooth.
4. Taste and adjust seasoning if needed.
5. Ladle the soup into bowls and garnish with fresh basil leaves, if desired. Serve with croutons on the side for added texture, if desired.
6. Serve hot and enjoy this classic and comforting tomato basil soup!

Nutritional Information (per serving):

- Calories: 120
- Protein: 3g
- Fat: 3g
- Carbohydrates: 20g
- Fiber: 5g

Chicken and Vegetable Soup

Prep Time: 15 mins

Total Time: 45 mins

Servings: 4

Ingredients:

- 1 tablespoon olive oil
- 1 onion, diced
- 2 cloves garlic, minced
- 2 carrots, diced
- 2 celery stalks, diced
- 1 medium potato, diced
- 4 cups low-sodium chicken broth
- 2 cups shredded cooked chicken breast
- 1 teaspoon dried thyme
- Salt and pepper to taste
- Fresh parsley for garnish (optional)

Directions:

1. In a large pot, heat olive oil over medium heat. Add diced onion and minced garlic, and sauté until softened, about 5 minutes.
2. Add diced carrots, celery, and potato to the pot, and cook for another 5 minutes until slightly softened.
3. Pour in the chicken broth and bring to a boil. Reduce heat to low, cover, and simmer for 20 minutes until vegetables are tender.
4. Stir in shredded cooked chicken breast and dried thyme. Simmer for another 10 minutes.

5. Season with salt and pepper to taste.
6. Ladle the soup into bowls, garnish with fresh parsley if desired, and serve hot.

Nutritional Information (per serving):
- Calories: 210
- Protein: 20g
- Fat: 6g
- Carbohydrates: 18g
- Fiber: 3g

Lentil and Spinach Soup

Prep Time: 10 mins

Total Time: 40 mins

Servings: 4

Ingredients:
- 1 tablespoon olive oil
- 1 onion, chopped
- 2 cloves garlic, minced
- 1 carrot, diced
- 1 celery stalk, diced
- 1 cup dried green lentils, rinsed
- 4 cups vegetable broth
- 2 cups fresh spinach leaves
- 1 teaspoon ground cumin
- Salt and pepper to taste
- Lemon wedges for serving (optional)

Directions:

1. Heat olive oil in a large pot over medium heat. Add chopped onion and minced garlic, and sauté until softened, about 5 minutes.
2. Add diced carrot and celery to the pot, and cook for another 5 minutes until slightly softened.
3. Stir in rinsed lentils, vegetable broth, and ground cumin. Bring to a boil, then reduce heat to low, cover, and simmer for 25 minutes until lentils are tender.
4. Add fresh spinach leaves to the pot and stir until wilted, about 3 minutes.
5. Season with salt and pepper to taste.
6. Serve the soup hot with lemon wedges on the side for squeezing over the soup if desired.

Nutritional Information (per serving):
- Calories: 240
- Protein: 13g
- Fat: 3g
- Carbohydrates: 40g
- Fiber: 17g

Butternut Squash Soup

Prep Time: 15 mins
Total Time: 45 mins
Servings: 4

Ingredients:
- 1 tablespoon olive oil
- 1 onion, chopped

- 2 cloves garlic, minced
- 1 butternut squash, peeled, seeded, and diced
- 2 carrots, chopped
- 4 cups vegetable broth
- 1 teaspoon ground cinnamon
- 1/2 teaspoon ground nutmeg
- Salt and pepper to taste
- Plain yogurt or coconut cream for garnish (optional)
- Fresh chives for garnish (optional)

Directions:

1. In a large pot, heat olive oil over medium heat. Add chopped onion and minced garlic, and sauté until softened, about 5 minutes.
2. Add diced butternut squash and chopped carrots to the pot, and cook for another 5 minutes until slightly softened.
3. Pour in vegetable broth and add ground cinnamon and ground nutmeg. Bring to a boil, then reduce heat to low, cover, and simmer for 25 minutes until vegetables are tender.
4. Use an immersion blender to puree the soup until smooth. Alternatively, transfer the soup to a blender and blend in batches until smooth.
5. Season with salt and pepper to taste.
6. Ladle the soup into bowls, and garnish with a dollop of plain yogurt or coconut cream and fresh chives if desired.

Nutritional Information (per serving):

- Calories: 180

- Protein: 3g
- Fat: 4g
- Carbohydrates: 35g
- Fiber: 7g

Mushroom Barley Soup

Prep Time: 15 mins

Total Time: 1 hour

Servings: 4

Ingredients:
- 1 tablespoon olive oil
- 1 onion, chopped
- 2 cloves garlic, minced
- 8 oz mushrooms, sliced (such as cremini or button mushrooms)
- 1 carrot, diced
- 1 celery stalk, diced
- 1/2 cup pearl barley, rinsed
- 4 cups vegetable broth
- 1 teaspoon dried thyme
- Salt and pepper to taste
- Fresh parsley for garnish (optional)

Directions:
1. Heat olive oil in a large pot over medium heat. Add chopped onion and minced garlic, and sauté until softened, about 5 minutes.

2. Add sliced mushrooms, diced carrot, and diced celery to the pot, and cook for another 5 minutes until mushrooms release their juices.
3. Stir in rinsed pearl barley, vegetable broth, and dried thyme. Bring to a boil, then reduce heat to low, cover, and simmer for 40 minutes until barley is tender.
4. Season with salt and pepper to taste.
5. Ladle the soup into bowls, and garnish with fresh parsley if desired.

Nutritional Information (per serving):
- Calories: 220
- Protein: 7g
- Fat: 4g
- Carbohydrates: 40g
- Fiber: 8g

Tomato and White Bean Soup

Prep Time: 10 mins

Total Time: 30 mins

Servings: 4

Ingredients:
- 1 tablespoon olive oil
- 1 onion, chopped
- 2 cloves garlic, minced
- 1 can (15 oz) diced tomatoes
- 2 cups vegetable broth
- 1 can (15 oz) cannellini beans, drained and rinsed

- 1 teaspoon dried basil
- 1/2 teaspoon dried oregano
- Salt and pepper to taste
- Fresh basil leaves for garnish (optional)
- Grated Parmesan cheese for garnish (optional)

Directions:

1. In a large pot, heat olive oil over medium heat. Add chopped onion and minced garlic, and sauté until softened, about 5 minutes.
2. Add diced tomatoes (with their juices) to the pot, along with vegetable broth, cannellini beans, dried basil, and dried oregano. Bring to a boil, then reduce heat to low, cover, and simmer for 15 minutes.
3. Use an immersion blender to partially blend the soup, leaving some chunks of tomatoes and beans for texture. Alternatively, transfer a portion of the soup to a blender and blend until smooth, then return it to the pot.
4. Season with salt and pepper to taste.
5. Ladle the soup into bowls, and garnish with fresh basil leaves and grated Parmesan cheese if desired.

Nutritional Information (per serving):

- Calories: 180
- Protein: 8g
- Fat: 4g
- Carbohydrates: 30g
- Fiber: 7g

SEAFOOD RECIPES

Grilled Lemon Herb Salmon

Prep Time: 10 mins

Total Time: 20 mins

Servings: 4

Ingredients:

- 4 salmon fillets (about 6 oz each)
- 2 tablespoons olive oil
- 2 cloves garlic, minced
- 1 tablespoon fresh lemon juice
- 1 teaspoon lemon zest
- 1 teaspoon chopped fresh thyme
- Salt and pepper to taste
- Lemon wedges for serving
- Fresh parsley for garnish (optional)

Directions:

1. Preheat grill to medium-high heat.
2. In a small bowl, mix together olive oil, minced garlic, lemon juice, lemon zest, and chopped thyme.
3. Brush both sides of the salmon fillets with the lemon herb mixture and season with salt and pepper.
4. Place the salmon fillets on the grill and cook for about 4-5 minutes per side, or until cooked through and flaky.
5. Remove from the grill and serve hot with lemon wedges. Garnish with fresh parsley if desired.

Nutritional Information (per serving):
- Calories: 300
- Protein: 34g
- Fat: 18g
- Carbohydrates: 1g
- Fiber: 0g

Baked Lemon Garlic Shrimp

Prep Time: 10 mins

Total Time: 20 mins

Servings: 4

Ingredients:
- 1 lb large shrimp, peeled and deveined
- 2 tablespoons olive oil
- 3 cloves garlic, minced
- 2 tablespoons fresh lemon juice
- 1 teaspoon lemon zest
- 1 teaspoon dried oregano
- Salt and pepper to taste
- Fresh parsley for garnish
- Lemon wedges for serving

Directions:
1. Preheat oven to 400°F (200°C).
2. In a large bowl, combine olive oil, minced garlic, lemon juice, lemon zest, dried oregano, salt, and pepper.
3. Add the shrimp to the bowl and toss until evenly coated.
4. Transfer the shrimp to a baking dish in a single layer.

5. Bake in the preheated oven for 8-10 minutes, or until the shrimp are pink and cooked through.
6. Remove from the oven, garnish with fresh parsley, and serve with lemon wedges.

Nutritional Information (per serving):
- Calories: 180
- Protein: 24g
- Fat: 8g
- Carbohydrates: 3g
- Fiber: 0g

Seared Scallops with Garlic Butter

Prep Time: 10 mins

Total Time: 15 mins

Servings: 4

Ingredients:
- 1 lb large sea scallops
- 2 tablespoons unsalted butter
- 2 cloves garlic, minced
- Salt and pepper to taste
- Fresh parsley for garnish
- Lemon wedges for serving

Directions:
1. Pat the scallops dry with paper towels and season with salt and pepper on both sides.
2. Heat a large skillet over medium-high heat and add butter.

3. Once the butter has melted, add minced garlic to the skillet and cook for about 1 minute until fragrant.
4. Add the scallops to the skillet in a single layer, making sure not to overcrowd the pan. Cook for 2-3 minutes per side, or until golden brown and caramelized.
5. Remove the scallops from the skillet and transfer to a serving plate.
6. Garnish with fresh parsley and serve immediately with lemon wedges.

Nutritional Information (per serving):
- Calories: 160
- Protein: 19g
- Fat: 8g
- Carbohydrates: 2g
- Fiber: 0g

Grilled Shrimp Skewers

Prep Time: 15 mins

Total Time: 20 mins

Servings: 4

Ingredients:
- 1 lb large shrimp, peeled and deveined
- 2 tablespoons olive oil
- 2 cloves garlic, minced
- 1 tablespoon fresh lemon juice
- 1 teaspoon lemon zest
- 1 teaspoon paprika

- Salt and pepper to taste
- Wooden skewers, soaked in water for 30 minutes
- Lemon wedges for serving
- Fresh parsley for garnish

Directions:
1. Preheat grill to medium-high heat.
2. In a large bowl, combine olive oil, minced garlic, lemon juice, lemon zest, paprika, salt, and pepper.
3. Add the shrimp to the bowl and toss until evenly coated.
4. Thread the shrimp onto the soaked wooden skewers.
5. Grill the shrimp skewers for 2-3 minutes per side, or until they are pink and cooked through.
6. Remove from the grill and serve hot with lemon wedges. Garnish with fresh parsley if desired.

Nutritional Information (per serving):
- Calories: 180
- Protein: 22g
- Fat: 9g
- Carbohydrates: 2g
- Fiber: 0g

Pan-Seared Halibut with Lemon Herb Sauce

Prep Time: 10 mins

Total Time: 20 mins

Servings: 4

Ingredients:
- 4 halibut fillets (about 6 oz each)

- Salt and pepper to taste
- 2 tablespoons olive oil
- 2 tablespoons unsalted butter
- 2 cloves garlic, minced
- 2 tablespoons fresh lemon juice
- 1 teaspoon lemon zest
- 1 tablespoon chopped fresh parsley
- 1 tablespoon chopped fresh dill

Directions:

1. Season the halibut fillets with salt and pepper on both sides.
2. Heat olive oil in a large skillet over medium-high heat.
3. Add the halibut fillets to the skillet and cook for 3-4 minutes per side, or until golden brown and cooked through.
4. Remove the halibut from the skillet and transfer to a serving plate.
5. In the same skillet, melt butter over medium heat. Add minced garlic and cook for 1 minute until fragrant.
6. Stir in fresh lemon juice, lemon zest, chopped parsley, and chopped dill. Cook for another minute, then remove from heat.
7. Spoon the lemon herb sauce over the pan-seared halibut fillets.
8. Serve immediately with your choice of side dishes.

Nutritional Information (per serving):

- Calories: 250
- Protein: 30g
- Fat: 14g
- Carbohydrates: 1g

- Fiber: 0g

These seafood recipes are not only delicious but also suitable for individuals following an EPI diet, providing essential nutrients while being gentle on the digestive system. Enjoy these flavorful dishes as part of a balanced diet.

Cajun Grilled Shrimp Tacos

Prep Time: 15 mins

Total Time: 25 mins

Servings: 4

Ingredients:

- 1 lb large shrimp, peeled and deveined
- 2 tablespoons olive oil
- 2 teaspoons Cajun seasoning
- Salt and pepper to taste
- 8 small corn tortillas
- 1 cup shredded cabbage
- 1 avocado, sliced
- 1/4 cup diced tomatoes
- 1/4 cup diced red onions
- Lime wedges for serving
- Fresh cilantro for garnish

Directions:

1. Preheat grill to medium-high heat.
2. In a bowl, toss the shrimp with olive oil, Cajun seasoning, salt, and pepper until evenly coated.
3. Thread the seasoned shrimp onto skewers.

4. Grill the shrimp skewers for 2-3 minutes per side, or until they are pink and cooked through.
5. Warm the corn tortillas on the grill for about 30 seconds per side.
6. To assemble the tacos, place a few shrimp on each tortilla and top with shredded cabbage, sliced avocado, diced tomatoes, and red onions.
7. Serve the tacos hot with lime wedges on the side for squeezing. Garnish with fresh cilantro.

Nutritional Information (per serving):
- Calories: 280
- Protein: 22g
- Fat: 12g
- Carbohydrates: 24g
- Fiber: 6g

Baked Lemon Garlic Cod

Prep Time: 10 mins

Total Time: 20 mins

Servings: 4

Ingredients:
- 4 cod fillets (about 6 oz each)
- 2 tablespoons olive oil
- 3 cloves garlic, minced
- 2 tablespoons fresh lemon juice
- 1 teaspoon lemon zest
- 1 teaspoon dried parsley

- Salt and pepper to taste
- Lemon wedges for serving
- Fresh parsley for garnish

Directions:
1. Preheat oven to 400°F (200°C).
2. Place the cod fillets on a baking sheet lined with parchment paper.
3. In a small bowl, whisk together olive oil, minced garlic, lemon juice, lemon zest, dried parsley, salt, and pepper.
4. Drizzle the lemon garlic mixture over the cod fillets.
5. Bake in the preheated oven for 12-15 minutes, or until the cod is opaque and flakes easily with a fork.
6. Remove from the oven and serve hot with lemon wedges. Garnish with fresh parsley.

Nutritional Information (per serving):
- Calories: 220
- Protein: 26g
- Fat: 10g
- Carbohydrates: 2g
- Fiber: 0g

Coconut Shrimp Curry

Prep Time: 15 mins

Total Time: 30 mins

Servings: 4

Ingredients:
- 1 lb large shrimp, peeled and deveined

- 2 tablespoons coconut oil
- 1 onion, diced
- 3 cloves garlic, minced
- 1 tablespoon grated ginger
- 2 tablespoons curry powder
- 1 teaspoon ground turmeric
- 1 can (14 oz) coconut milk
- 1 cup vegetable broth
- 1 tablespoon fish sauce
- 2 cups fresh spinach
- Salt and pepper to taste
- Cooked rice for serving

Directions:

1. In a large skillet, heat coconut oil over medium heat. Add diced onion and cook until softened.
2. Add minced garlic and grated ginger to the skillet and cook for 1 minute until fragrant.
3. Stir in curry powder and ground turmeric, and cook for another minute.
4. Pour in coconut milk, vegetable broth, and fish sauce. Bring to a simmer.
5. Add shrimp to the skillet and cook for 5-7 minutes, or until the shrimp are pink and cooked through.
6. Stir in fresh spinach and cook until wilted. Season with salt and pepper to taste.
7. Serve the coconut shrimp curry hot over cooked rice.

Nutritional Information (per serving):
- Calories: 320
- Protein: 24g
- Fat: 21g
- Carbohydrates: 15g
- Fiber: 2g

Lemon Garlic Butter Scallops

Prep Time: 10 mins

Total Time: 15 mins

Servings: 4

Ingredients:
- 1 lb large sea scallops
- Salt and pepper to taste
- 2 tablespoons unsalted butter
- 3 cloves garlic, minced
- 2 tablespoons fresh lemon juice
- 1 teaspoon lemon zest
- 1 tablespoon chopped fresh parsley

Directions:
1. Pat the scallops dry with paper towels and season with salt and pepper on both sides.
2. Heat a large skillet over medium-high heat and add butter.
3. Once the butter has melted, add minced garlic to the skillet and cook for 1 minute until fragrant.

4. Add the scallops to the skillet in a single layer and cook for 2-3 minutes per side, or until they are golden brown and opaque in the center.
5. Drizzle fresh lemon juice over the scallops and sprinkle with lemon zest and chopped parsley.
6. Remove from heat and serve the lemon garlic butter scallops immediately.

Nutritional Information (per serving):
- Calories: 180
- Protein: 20g
- Fat: 9g
- Carbohydrates: 4g
- Fiber: 0g

Grilled Salmon with Dill Sauce

Prep Time: 10 mins
Total Time: 20 mins
Servings: 4

Ingredients:
- 4 salmon fillets (about 6 oz each)
- 2 tablespoons olive oil
- Salt and pepper to taste
- 1/4 cup Greek yogurt
- 2 tablespoons chopped fresh dill
- 1 tablespoon lemon juice
- 1 teaspoon lemon zest
- 1 clove garlic, minced

Directions:
1. Preheat grill to medium-high heat.
2. Brush salmon fillets with olive oil and season with salt and pepper.
3. Grill the salmon fillets for 4-5 minutes per side, or until they are cooked through and flake easily with a fork.
4. In a small bowl, mix together Greek yogurt, chopped fresh dill, lemon juice, lemon zest, and minced garlic to make the dill sauce.
5. Serve the grilled salmon hot with a dollop of dill sauce on top.

Nutritional Information (per serving):
- Calories: 320
- Protein: 28g
- Fat: 20g
- Carbohydrates: 2g
- Fiber: 0g

Grilled Lemon Herb Salmon

Prep Time: 10 mins

Total Time: 20 mins

Servings: 4

Ingredients:
- 4 salmon fillets (6 oz each)
- 2 tablespoons olive oil
- 2 cloves garlic, minced
- 1 tablespoon fresh lemon juice
- 1 teaspoon lemon zest

- 1 teaspoon chopped fresh thyme
- Salt and pepper to taste
- Lemon wedges for serving
- Fresh parsley for garnish

Directions:
1. Preheat grill to medium-high heat.
2. In a small bowl, whisk together olive oil, minced garlic, lemon juice, lemon zest, chopped thyme, salt, and pepper.
3. Brush the mixture over the salmon fillets, coating evenly.
4. Place the salmon fillets on the grill and cook for 4-5 minutes per side, or until the fish flakes easily with a fork.
5. Remove from the grill and serve hot with lemon wedges. Garnish with fresh parsley.

Nutritional Information (per serving):
- Calories: 300
- Protein: 28g
- Fat: 18g
- Carbohydrates: 2g
- Fiber: 0g

Lemon Garlic Shrimp Pasta

Prep Time: 15 mins

Total Time: 25 mins

Servings: 4

Ingredients:
- 8 oz whole wheat pasta
- 1 lb large shrimp, peeled and deveined

- 2 tablespoons olive oil
- 4 cloves garlic, minced
- 2 tablespoons fresh lemon juice
- 1 teaspoon lemon zest
- 1/4 cup chopped fresh parsley
- Salt and pepper to taste
- Grated Parmesan cheese for serving

Directions:

1. Cook the pasta according to package instructions until al dente. Drain and set aside.
2. In a large skillet, heat olive oil over medium heat. Add minced garlic and cook until fragrant.
3. Add the shrimp to the skillet and cook for 2-3 minutes per side, or until pink and cooked through.
4. Stir in fresh lemon juice, lemon zest, chopped parsley, salt, and pepper.
5. Add the cooked pasta to the skillet and toss until well coated with the shrimp and sauce.
6. Serve hot with grated Parmesan cheese on top.

Nutritional Information (per serving):

- Calories: 380
- Protein: 30g
- Fat: 10g
- Carbohydrates: 40g
- Fiber: 6g

Baked Lemon Dill Cod

Prep Time: 10 mins

Total Time: 20 mins

Servings: 4

Ingredients:

- 4 cod fillets (6 oz each)
- 2 tablespoons olive oil
- 2 cloves garlic, minced
- 2 tablespoons fresh lemon juice
- 1 teaspoon lemon zest
- 1 tablespoon chopped fresh dill
- Salt and pepper to taste
- Lemon wedges for serving

Directions:

1. Preheat oven to 400°F (200°C).
2. Place the cod fillets on a baking sheet lined with parchment paper.
3. In a small bowl, whisk together olive oil, minced garlic, lemon juice, lemon zest, chopped dill, salt, and pepper.
4. Brush the mixture over the cod fillets, coating evenly.
5. Bake in the preheated oven for 12-15 minutes, or until the fish is opaque and flakes easily with a fork.
6. Serve hot with lemon wedges on the side.

Nutritional Information (per serving):

- Calories: 240
- Protein: 30g
- Fat: 10g

- Carbohydrates: 2g
- Fiber: 0g

Garlic Butter Scallops

Prep Time: 10 mins

Total Time: 15 mins

Servings: 4

Ingredients:

- 1 lb large sea scallops
- 2 tablespoons unsalted butter
- 2 cloves garlic, minced
- 1 tablespoon chopped fresh parsley
- Salt and pepper to taste
- Lemon wedges for serving

Directions:

1. Pat the scallops dry with paper towels and season with salt and pepper.
2. Heat a large skillet over medium-high heat and add butter.
3. Once the butter has melted, add minced garlic to the skillet and cook for 1 minute until fragrant.
4. Add the scallops to the skillet in a single layer and cook for 2-3 minutes per side, or until they are golden brown and opaque in the center.
5. Sprinkle chopped fresh parsley over the scallops and serve hot with lemon wedges.

Nutritional Information (per serving):

- Calories: 160

- Protein: 20g
- Fat: 8g
- Carbohydrates: 2g
- Fiber: 0g

Lemon Herb Tilapia

Prep Time: 10 mins

Total Time: 20 mins

Servings: 4

Ingredients:

- 4 tilapia fillets (6 oz each)
- 2 tablespoons olive oil
- 2 cloves garlic, minced
- 2 tablespoons fresh lemon juice
- 1 teaspoon lemon zest
- 1 tablespoon chopped fresh parsley
- Salt and pepper to taste

Directions:

1. Preheat oven to 400°F (200°C).
2. Place the tilapia fillets on a baking sheet lined with parchment paper.
3. In a small bowl, whisk together olive oil, minced garlic, lemon juice, lemon zest, chopped parsley, salt, and pepper.
4. Brush the mixture over the tilapia fillets, coating evenly.
5. Bake in the preheated oven for 12-15 minutes, or until the fish is opaque and flakes easily with a fork.
6. Serve hot with additional lemon wedges if desired.

Nutritional Information (per serving):

- Calories: 180
- Protein: 26g
- Fat: 8g
- Carbohydrates: 2g
- Fiber: 0g

Lemon Garlic Grilled Shrimp

Prep Time: 10 mins

Total Time: 15 mins

Servings: 4

Ingredients:

- 1 lb large shrimp, peeled and deveined
- 2 cloves garlic, minced
- 2 tablespoons olive oil
- 1 tablespoon fresh lemon juice
- 1 teaspoon lemon zest
- 1 teaspoon chopped fresh parsley
- Salt and pepper to taste
- Lemon wedges for serving

Directions:

1. Preheat grill to medium-high heat.
2. In a bowl, combine minced garlic, olive oil, lemon juice, lemon zest, chopped parsley, salt, and pepper.
3. Add the shrimp to the bowl and toss until evenly coated.
4. Thread the shrimp onto skewers.

5. Grill the shrimp for 2-3 minutes per side until pink and cooked through.
   6. Serve hot with lemon wedges on the side.

Nutritional Information (per serving):
- Calories: 180
- Protein: 25g
- Fat: 8g
- Carbohydrates: 2g
- Fiber: 0g

Baked Salmon with Dill

Prep Time: 10 mins

Total Time: 20 mins

Servings: 4

Ingredients:
- 4 salmon fillets (6 oz each)
- 2 tablespoons olive oil
- 2 cloves garlic, minced
- 1 tablespoon fresh lemon juice
- 1 teaspoon lemon zest
- 1 tablespoon chopped fresh dill
- Salt and pepper to taste
- Lemon wedges for serving

Directions:
   1. Preheat oven to 400°F (200°C).
   2. Place the salmon fillets on a baking sheet lined with parchment paper.

3. In a bowl, whisk together olive oil, minced garlic, lemon juice, lemon zest, chopped dill, salt, and pepper.
4. Brush the mixture over the salmon fillets, coating evenly.
5. Bake in the preheated oven for 12-15 minutes until the salmon flakes easily with a fork.
6. Serve hot with lemon wedges on the side.

Nutritional Information (per serving):
- Calories: 320
- Protein: 35g
- Fat: 18g
- Carbohydrates: 2g
- Fiber: 0g

Garlic Butter Lobster Tails

- **Prep Time:** 10 mins
- **Total Time:** 20 mins
- **Servings:** 4

Ingredients:
- 4 lobster tails
- 4 tablespoons unsalted butter
- 4 cloves garlic, minced
- 1 tablespoon chopped fresh parsley
- Salt and pepper to taste
- Lemon wedges for serving

Directions:
1. Preheat oven to 375°F (190°C).

2. Use kitchen shears to cut the top of each lobster tail shell lengthwise.
3. In a microwave-safe bowl, melt the butter and stir in minced garlic and chopped parsley.
4. Brush the garlic butter mixture over the lobster tails.
5. Place the lobster tails on a baking sheet and bake for 12-15 minutes until the lobster meat is opaque and white.
6. Serve hot with lemon wedges on the side.

Nutritional Information (per serving):
- Calories: 230
- Protein: 25g
- Fat: 14g
- Carbohydrates: 1g
- Fiber: 0g

Tuna Salad Lettuce Wraps

Prep Time: 15 mins
Total Time: 15 mins
Servings: 4

Ingredients:
- 2 cans (5 oz each) tuna, drained
- 1/4 cup mayonnaise
- 2 tablespoons chopped celery
- 2 tablespoons chopped red onion
- 1 tablespoon lemon juice
- Salt and pepper to taste
- Lettuce leaves for wrapping

Directions:
1. In a bowl, combine drained tuna, mayonnaise, chopped celery, chopped red onion, lemon juice, salt, and pepper.
2. Mix until well combined.
3. Spoon the tuna salad onto lettuce leaves.
4. Wrap the lettuce around the filling to form wraps.
5. Serve immediately.

Nutritional Information (per serving):
- Calories: 180
- Protein: 20g
- Fat: 10g
- Carbohydrates: 2g
- Fiber: 1g

Grilled Swordfish with Mango Salsa

Prep Time: 15 mins

Total Time: 25 mins

Servings: 4

Ingredients:
- 4 swordfish steaks (6 oz each)
- 2 tablespoons olive oil
- Salt and pepper to taste

Mango Salsa:
- 1 mango, peeled and diced
- 1/4 cup diced red bell pepper
- 2 tablespoons chopped fresh cilantro
- 1 tablespoon lime juice

- 1 tablespoon finely chopped red onion
- Salt and pepper to taste

Directions:
1. Preheat grill to medium-high heat.
2. Rub swordfish steaks with olive oil and season with salt and pepper.
3. Grill swordfish for 4-5 minutes per side until cooked through and grill marks appear.
4. In a bowl, combine diced mango, diced red bell pepper, chopped cilantro, lime juice, chopped red onion, salt, and pepper to make the salsa.
5. Serve grilled swordfish topped with mango salsa.

Nutritional Information (per serving):
- Calories: 280
- Protein: 30g
- Fat: 10g
- Carbohydrates: 15g
- Fiber: 2g

SMOOTHIE RECIPES

Berry Blast Smoothie

Prep Time: 5 mins

Total Time: 5 mins

Servings: 2 glasses

Ingredients:
- 1 cup frozen mixed berries (strawberries, blueberries, raspberries)
- 1/2 cup spinach leaves
- 1/2 ripe banana
- 1/2 cup unsweetened almond milk
- 1/2 cup plain Greek yogurt
- 1 tablespoon chia seeds
- 1 teaspoon honey (optional)

Directions:
1. Place all ingredients in a blender.
2. Blend until smooth and creamy.
3. If the consistency is too thick, add more almond milk.
4. Pour into glasses and serve immediately.

Nutritional Information (per serving):
- Calories: 150
- Protein: 8g
- Fat: 4g
- Carbohydrates: 23g
- Fiber: 6g

Tropical Paradise Smoothie

Prep Time: 5 mins

Total Time: 5 mins

Servings: 2 glasses

Ingredients:

- 1 cup frozen mango chunks
- 1/2 cup pineapple chunks
- 1/2 ripe banana
- 1/2 cup spinach leaves
- 1/2 cup coconut water
- 1/2 cup plain Greek yogurt
- 1 tablespoon shredded coconut

Directions:

1. Combine all ingredients in a blender.
2. Blend until smooth.
3. Add more coconut water if needed to reach desired consistency.
4. Pour into glasses and garnish with shredded coconut if desired.

Nutritional Information (per serving):

- Calories: 180
- Protein: 8g
- Fat: 3g
- Carbohydrates: 34g
- Fiber: 6g

Green Goddess Smoothie

Prep Time: 5 mins

Total Time: 5 mins

Servings: 2 glasses

Ingredients:

- 1 cup fresh spinach
- 1/2 ripe avocado
- 1/2 cucumber, peeled and chopped
- 1/2 cup coconut water
- 1/2 cup plain Greek yogurt
- Juice of 1/2 lime
- 1 tablespoon fresh mint leaves
- 1 teaspoon honey (optional)

Directions:

1. Combine all ingredients in a blender.
2. Blend until smooth and creamy.
3. Adjust sweetness with honey if desired.
4. Pour into glasses and serve immediately.

Nutritional Information (per serving):

- Calories: 160
- Protein: 8g
- Fat: 7g
- Carbohydrates: 18g
- Fiber: 6g

Protein Power Smoothie

Prep Time: 5 mins

Total Time: 5 mins

Servings: 2 glasses

Ingredients:

- 1 cup unsweetened almond milk
- 1/2 cup plain Greek yogurt
- 1 scoop vanilla protein powder
- 1/2 cup frozen strawberries
- 1/2 ripe banana
- 1 tablespoon almond butter
- 1 teaspoon honey (optional)

Directions:
1. Add all ingredients to a blender.
2. Blend until smooth and creamy.
3. Adjust sweetness with honey if needed.
4. Pour into glasses and enjoy immediately.

Nutritional Information (per serving):
- Calories: 240
- Protein: 25g
- Fat: 7g
- Carbohydrates: 20g
- Fiber: 4g

Coconut Kale Smoothie

Prep Time: 5 mins

Total Time: 5 mins

Servings: 2 glasses

Ingredients:
- 1 cup coconut water
- 1/2 cup coconut milk
- 1 cup kale leaves, stems removed

- 1/2 cup frozen pineapple chunks
- 1/2 frozen banana
- 1 tablespoon unsweetened shredded coconut

Directions:
1. Combine all ingredients in a blender.
2. Blend until smooth and creamy.
3. Add more coconut water if necessary to reach desired consistency.
4. Pour into glasses and serve immediately.

Nutritional Information (per serving):
- Calories: 150
- Protein: 3g
- Fat: 8g
- Carbohydrates: 20g
- Fiber: 4g

Tropical Green Smoothie

Prep Time: 5 mins

Total Time: 5 mins

Servings: 2 glasses

Ingredients:
- 1 cup frozen mango chunks
- 1/2 cup frozen pineapple chunks
- 1 cup spinach leaves
- 1/2 ripe banana
- 1 cup coconut water
- 1 tablespoon chia seeds

Directions:

1. Combine all ingredients in a blender.
2. Blend until smooth and creamy.
3. Add more coconut water if needed for desired consistency.
4. Pour into glasses and serve immediately.

Nutritional Information (per serving):

- Calories: 180
- Protein: 5g
- Fat: 5g
- Carbohydrates: 32g
- Fiber: 7g

Berry Spinach Smoothie

Prep Time: 5 mins

Total Time: 5 mins

Servings: 2 glasses

Ingredients:

- 1 cup frozen mixed berries (strawberries, blueberries, raspberries)
- 1 cup spinach leaves
- 1/2 ripe banana
- 1/2 cup almond milk
- 1 tablespoon flaxseeds
- 1 tablespoon honey (optional)

Directions:

1. Place all ingredients in a blender.
2. Blend until smooth.

3. Add more almond milk if necessary to reach desired consistency.
4. Pour into glasses and serve immediately.

Nutritional Information (per serving):
- Calories: 160
- Protein: 4g
- Fat: 4g
- Carbohydrates: 30g
- Fiber: 7g

Creamy Avocado Smoothie

Prep Time: 5 mins
Total Time: 5 mins
Servings: 2 glasses

Ingredients:
- 1/2 avocado
- 1 cup spinach leaves
- 1/2 cucumber, peeled and chopped
- 1/2 cup coconut water
- Juice of 1/2 lime
- 1 tablespoon fresh mint leaves
- 1 teaspoon agave nectar (optional)

Directions:
1. Combine all ingredients in a blender.
2. Blend until smooth and creamy.
3. Adjust sweetness with agave nectar if desired.
4. Pour into glasses and serve immediately.

Nutritional Information (per serving):
- Calories: 120
- Protein: 3g
- Fat: 7g
- Carbohydrates: 14g
- Fiber: 6g

Peanut Butter Banana Smoothie

Prep Time: 5 mins

Total Time: 5 mins

Servings: 2 glasses

Ingredients:
- 1 ripe banana
- 2 tablespoons natural peanut butter
- 1 cup spinach leaves
- 1 cup unsweetened almond milk
- 1 tablespoon chia seeds
- 1 tablespoon honey (optional)

Directions:
1. Combine all ingredients in a blender.
2. Blend until smooth and creamy.
3. Add more almond milk if needed to reach desired consistency.
4. Pour into glasses and serve immediately.

Nutritional Information (per serving):
- Calories: 250
- Protein: 8g
- Fat: 15g

- Carbohydrates: 25g
- Fiber: 7g

Blueberry Almond Smoothie

Prep Time: 5 mins

Total Time: 5 mins

Servings: 2 glasses

Ingredients:
- 1 cup frozen blueberries
- 1 cup spinach leaves
- 1/2 cup almond milk
- 1/4 cup plain Greek yogurt
- 2 tablespoons almond butter
- 1 tablespoon honey (optional)

Directions:
1. Place all ingredients in a blender.
2. Blend until smooth and creamy.
3. Adjust sweetness with honey if desired.
4. Pour into glasses and serve immediately.

Nutritional Information (per serving):
- Calories: 230
- Protein: 8g
- Fat: 12g
- Carbohydrates: 25g
- Fiber: 6g

Berry Blast Smoothie

Prep Time: 5 mins

Total Time: 5 mins

Servings: 2 glasses

Ingredients:

- 1 cup frozen mixed berries (strawberries, blueberries, raspberries)
- 1/2 cup spinach leaves
- 1/2 ripe banana
- 1 cup almond milk
- 1 tablespoon chia seeds
- 1 teaspoon honey (optional)

Directions:

1. Place all ingredients in a blender.
2. Blend until smooth.
3. Add more almond milk if necessary to reach desired consistency.
4. Pour into glasses and serve immediately.

Nutritional Information (per serving):

- Calories: 180
- Protein: 4g
- Fat: 5g
- Carbohydrates: 30g
- Fiber: 8g

Green Goddess Smoothie

Prep Time: 5 mins

Total Time: 5 mins

Servings: 2 glasses

Ingredients:

- 1 cup spinach leaves
- 1/2 avocado
- 1/2 cucumber, peeled and chopped
- 1/2 cup coconut water
- Juice of 1/2 lime
- 1 tablespoon fresh mint leaves
- 1 teaspoon agave nectar (optional)

Directions:

1. Combine all ingredients in a blender.
2. Blend until smooth and creamy.
3. Adjust sweetness with agave nectar if desired.
4. Pour into glasses and serve immediately.

Nutritional Information (per serving):

- Calories: 120
- Protein: 3g
- Fat: 7g
- Carbohydrates: 14g
- Fiber: 6g

Tropical Paradise Smoothie

Prep Time: 5 mins

Total Time: 5 mins

Servings: 2 glasses

Ingredients:

- 1 cup frozen pineapple chunks

- 1/2 cup frozen mango chunks
- 1 cup spinach leaves
- 1/2 banana
- 1/2 cup coconut milk
- 1 tablespoon flaxseeds

Directions:
1. Combine all ingredients in a blender.
2. Blend until smooth.
3. Add more coconut milk if necessary for desired consistency.
4. Pour into glasses and serve immediately.

Nutritional Information (per serving):
- Calories: 200
- Protein: 4g
- Fat: 8g
- Carbohydrates: 30g
- Fiber: 6g

Creamy Berry Smoothie

Prep Time: 5 mins

Total Time: 5 mins

Servings: 2 glasses

Ingredients:
- 1 cup mixed frozen berries
- 1/2 cup Greek yogurt
- 1/2 cup almond milk
- 1 tablespoon almond butter
- 1 tablespoon honey (optional)

Directions:

1. Place all ingredients in a blender.
2. Blend until smooth and creamy.
3. Adjust sweetness with honey if desired.
4. Pour into glasses and serve immediately.

Nutritional Information (per serving):

- Calories: 230
- Protein: 9g
- Fat: 10g
- Carbohydrates: 29g
- Fiber: 6g

Chocolate Peanut Butter Smoothie

Prep Time: 5 mins

Total Time: 5 mins

Servings: 2 glasses

Ingredients:

- 1 ripe banana
- 2 tablespoons natural peanut butter
- 1 tablespoon cocoa powder
- 1 cup almond milk
- 1 tablespoon honey (optional)

Directions:

1. Combine all ingredients in a blender.
2. Blend until smooth and creamy.
3. Add more almond milk if needed to reach desired consistency.
4. Pour into glasses and serve immediately.

Nutritional Information (per serving):
- Calories: 280
- Protein: 8g
- Fat: 15g
- Carbohydrates: 33g
- Fiber: 7g

Green Detox Smoothie

Prep Time: 5 mins
Total Time: 5 mins
Servings: 2 glasses

Ingredients:
- 1 cup spinach
- 1/2 cup kale
- 1/2 cucumber, chopped
- 1/2 green apple, chopped
- 1/2 avocado
- Juice of 1 lemon
- 1 cup coconut water
- 1 tablespoon chia seeds
- Optional: 1 teaspoon honey or agave nectar

Directions:
1. Combine all ingredients in a blender.
2. Blend until smooth and creamy.
3. Taste and adjust sweetness with honey or agave nectar if desired.
4. Pour into glasses and serve immediately.

Nutritional Information (per serving):
- Calories: 150
- Protein: 5g
- Fat: 8g
- Carbohydrates: 18g
- Fiber: 7g

Berry Blast Smoothie

Prep Time: 5 mins
Total Time: 5 mins
Servings: 2 glasses

Ingredients:
- 1 cup frozen mixed berries (strawberries, blueberries, raspberries)
- 1/2 banana
- 1/2 cup spinach
- 1/2 cup almond milk
- 1 tablespoon flaxseeds
- Optional: 1 teaspoon honey or maple syrup

Directions:
1. Combine all ingredients in a blender.
2. Blend until smooth.
3. Adjust sweetness with honey or maple syrup if needed.
4. Pour into glasses and serve immediately.

Nutritional Information (per serving):
- Calories: 160
- Protein: 4g

- Fat: 6g
- Carbohydrates: 25g
- Fiber: 7g

Tropical Paradise Smoothie

Prep Time: 5 mins

Total Time: 5 mins

Servings: 2 glasses

Ingredients:
- 1/2 cup frozen pineapple chunks
- 1/2 cup frozen mango chunks
- 1/2 banana
- 1/2 cup coconut milk
- 1/2 cup spinach
- 1 tablespoon hemp seeds
- Optional: 1 teaspoon honey or agave nectar

Directions:
1. Combine all ingredients in a blender.
2. Blend until smooth.
3. Add honey or agave nectar for sweetness if desired.
4. Pour into glasses and serve immediately.

Nutritional Information (per serving):
- Calories: 220
- Protein: 4g
- Fat: 11g
- Carbohydrates: 29g
- Fiber: 5g

Creamy Peanut Butter Banana Smoothie

Prep Time: 5 mins

Total Time: 5 mins

Servings: 2 glasses

Ingredients:
- 1 banana
- 2 tablespoons natural peanut butter
- 1 cup almond milk
- 1/2 cup spinach
- 1 tablespoon chia seeds
- Optional: 1 teaspoon honey or maple syrup

Directions:
1. Combine all ingredients in a blender.
2. Blend until smooth and creamy.
3. Sweeten with honey or maple syrup if desired.
4. Pour into glasses and serve immediately.

Nutritional Information (per serving):
- Calories: 270
- Protein: 8g
- Fat: 15g
- Carbohydrates: 27g
- Fiber: 7g

Vanilla Almond Protein Smoothie

Prep Time: 5 mins

Total Time: 5 mins

Servings: 2 glasses

Ingredients:

- 1 cup unsweetened almond milk
- 1 scoop vanilla protein powder
- 1/2 banana
- 1 tablespoon almond butter
- 1/2 cup spinach
- Optional: 1 teaspoon honey or maple syrup

Directions:

1. Combine all ingredients in a blender.
2. Blend until smooth.
3. Sweeten with honey or maple syrup if desired.
4. Pour into glasses and serve immediately.

Nutritional Information (per serving):

- Calories: 240
- Protein: 22g
- Fat: 10g
- Carbohydrates: 17g
- Fiber: 4g

MEAL PLAN

Day 1
- **Breakfast:** Green Detox Smoothie
- **Lunch:** Berry Blast Smoothie
- **Dinner:** Grilled chicken with steamed vegetables

Day 2
- **Breakfast:** Tropical Paradise Smoothie
- **Lunch:** Creamy Peanut Butter Banana Smoothie
- **Dinner:** Baked salmon with quinoa and roasted vegetables

Day 3
- **Breakfast:** Vanilla Almond Protein Smoothie
- **Lunch:** Green Detox Smoothie
- **Dinner:** Stir-fried tofu with brown rice and mixed greens salad

Day 4
- **Breakfast:** Berry Blast Smoothie
- **Lunch:** Tropical Paradise Smoothie
- **Dinner:** Grilled shrimp skewers with cauliflower rice and sautéed spinach

Day 5
- **Breakfast:** Creamy Peanut Butter Banana Smoothie
- **Lunch:** Vanilla Almond Protein Smoothie
- **Dinner:** Baked chicken breast with sweet potato mash and steamed broccoli

Day 6
- **Breakfast:** Green Detox Smoothie
- **Lunch:** Berry Blast Smoothie
- **Dinner:** Pan-seared tilapia with quinoa pilaf and roasted asparagus

Day 7
- **Breakfast:** Tropical Paradise Smoothie
- **Lunch:** Creamy Peanut Butter Banana Smoothie
- **Dinner:** Vegetarian chili with cornbread and mixed greens salad

Day 8
- **Breakfast:** Vanilla Almond Protein Smoothie
- **Lunch:** Green Detox Smoothie
- **Dinner:** Grilled steak with roasted potatoes and sautéed kale

Day 9
- **Breakfast:** Berry Blast Smoothie
- **Lunch:** Tropical Paradise Smoothie
- **Dinner:** Baked cod with wild rice and steamed green beans

Day 10
- **Breakfast:** Creamy Peanut Butter Banana Smoothie
- **Lunch:** Vanilla Almond Protein Smoothie
- **Dinner:** Vegetable stir-fry with tofu and brown rice

Day 11
- **Breakfast:** Green Detox Smoothie

- **Lunch:** Berry Blast Smoothie
- **Dinner:** Grilled chicken Caesar salad with whole grain croutons

Day 12

- **Breakfast:** Tropical Paradise Smoothie
- **Lunch:** Creamy Peanut Butter Banana Smoothie
- **Dinner:** Baked salmon with quinoa tabbouleh and roasted carrots

Day 13

- **Breakfast:** Vanilla Almond Protein Smoothie
- **Lunch:** Green Detox Smoothie
- **Dinner:** Lentil soup with whole wheat bread and mixed greens salad

Day 14

- **Breakfast:** Berry Blast Smoothie
- **Lunch:** Tropical Paradise Smoothie
- **Dinner:** Spaghetti squash with marinara sauce and turkey meatballs

Day 15

- **Breakfast:** Creamy Peanut Butter Banana Smoothie
- **Lunch:** Vanilla Almond Protein Smoothie
- **Dinner:** Grilled shrimp tacos with avocado salsa and black bean salad

Day 16

- **Breakfast:** Green Detox Smoothie

- **Lunch:** Berry Blast Smoothie
- **Dinner:** Baked chicken thighs with sweet potato fries and steamed broccoli

Day 17

- **Breakfast:** Tropical Paradise Smoothie
- **Lunch:** Creamy Peanut Butter Banana Smoothie
- **Dinner:** Quinoa stuffed bell peppers with side salad

Day 18

- **Breakfast:** Vanilla Almond Protein Smoothie
- **Lunch:** Green Detox Smoothie
- Dinner: Beef and vegetable kebabs with couscous

Day 19

- **Breakfast:** Berry Blast Smoothie
- **Lunch:** Tropical Paradise Smoothie
- **Dinner:** Baked tilapia with wild rice pilaf and roasted Brussels sprouts

Day 20

- **Breakfast:** Creamy Peanut Butter Banana Smoothie
- **Lunch:** Vanilla Almond Protein Smoothie
- **Dinner:** Vegetarian lasagna with garlic bread and Caesar salad

Day 21

- **Breakfast:** Green Detox Smoothie
- **Lunch:** Berry Blast Smoothie

- **Dinner:** Grilled steak salad with mixed greens, tomatoes, and balsamic vinaigrette

CONCLUSION

In conclusion, the journey we've embarked upon through various recipes tailored for individuals with EPI (Exocrine Pancreatic Insufficiency) has been an enlightening exploration of nutrition, health, and wellness. By focusing on ingredients that are easily digestible and nutrient-rich, we've created a diverse array of meals that cater to the specific needs of those managing EPI while ensuring they are both delicious and satisfying.

Throughout this culinary adventure, we've discovered the importance of balance in our diets. From nutrient-packed smoothies bursting with antioxidants and vitamins to hearty soups and seafood dishes rich in protein and omega-3 fatty acids, each recipe has been carefully crafted to nourish the body and support overall well-being. By incorporating a variety of fruits, vegetables, lean proteins, and healthy fats, we've created meals that not only taste good but also provide essential nutrients vital for optimal health.

Moreover, we've emphasized the significance of mindful eating and listening to our bodies. By paying attention to how different foods make us feel and adjusting our diets accordingly, we can better manage symptoms associated with EPI and promote digestive health. From choosing whole, unprocessed foods to experimenting with herbs and spices for added flavor, we've demonstrated that eating well can be both enjoyable and beneficial.

Additionally, our exploration of cooking techniques and meal planning strategies has empowered us to make healthier choices in the kitchen. Whether it's grilling, baking, or sautéing, we've learned how to prepare nutritious meals without sacrificing taste or convenience. By taking the time to plan ahead and stock our pantries with wholesome ingredients, we've set ourselves up for success in maintaining a balanced diet that supports our health goals.

As we reflect on our culinary journey, let us remember the words of renowned chef and advocate for healthy living, Jamie Oliver: "The food you eat can be either the safest and most powerful form of medicine or the slowest form of poison." Indeed, our choices in the kitchen have a profound impact on our health and well-being. By prioritizing nutritious, EPI-friendly meals, we can nourish our bodies from the inside out and enjoy a vibrant, fulfilling life.

So let us continue to explore, experiment, and savor the joys of cooking with a renewed sense of purpose and dedication to our health. With each delicious meal we create, we take a step closer to achieving our wellness goals and living our best lives. Remember, the power to transform our health lies in our hands and on our plates.

In the words of Hippocrates, the father of modern medicine, "Let food be thy medicine and medicine be thy food." Let us embrace this wisdom and embark on a journey of self-discovery and healing through the transformative power of food. As we nourish our bodies with wholesome, EPI-friendly meals, may we also nourish our souls with the joy and vitality that comes from living well.

So here's to health, happiness, and delicious meals shared with loved ones. Cheers to a life filled with abundance, vitality, and the endless possibilities that come from taking care of ourselves—one meal at a time.

www.ingramcontent.com/pod-product-compliance
Lightning Source LLC
Chambersburg PA
CBHW052158220526
45471CB00004B/1728